Drugs for Medical Management of Obesity

Shilpa Chugh Garcha • Sanjay Kalra
Editors

Drugs for Medical Management of Obesity

A Machine-Generated Literature Overview

Springer

Editors
Shilpa Chugh Garcha
Sonepat, Haryana, India

Sanjay Kalra
Department of Endocrinology
Bharti Hospital
Karnal, Haryana, India

ISBN 978-981-96-1650-3 ISBN 978-981-96-1651-0 (eBook)
https://doi.org/10.1007/978-981-96-1651-0

This Springer imprint is published by the registered company Springer Nature Singapore Pte Ltd.
The registered company address is: 152 Beach Road, #21-01/04 Gateway East, Singapore 189721, Singapore

Preface

In the fast-evolving era of research and development in healthcare, last two decades have seen tremendous advancements and breakthroughs in newer innovative molecules in the field of obesity. A deeper understanding of the pathophysiology of obesity, its association with various comorbidities, and constant challenges in its management has led to an increased interest in this therapeutic area. Significant changes have been seen in the management of obesity over the last few years. Recently many medications have been approved by the regulatory authorities and a long list of newer molecules is in the clinical trial phase awaiting their use as anti-obesity medications.

This book is a machine-generated literature review of the anti-obesity medications that is written with an aim to provide an overview of their current scenario and various pipeline molecules that are in different stages of development. Machine generated summaries of various articles ranging from meta-analysis, clinical trials, and review articles to some case reports being published in the last few years are compiled and further organized into chapters. Each chapter has an introduction that provides the reader with a basis for further exploration of the topic. The chapters cover medications ranging from peripherally acting lipase inhibitors to fixed combination drugs to newer incretin mimetics and in one chapter we have also discussed the future developments in the management of obesity.

The book is intended for healthcare professionals, researchers, students, and anyone who is interested in the management of obesity, and innovative research molecules and future perspectives of anti-obesity medications. We encourage you to navigate through this book, and we hope that as a reader this book will help you have a better understanding of this rapidly advancing therapeutic area.

Sonepat, Haryana, India — Shilpa Chugh Garcha
Karnal, Haryana, India — Sanjay Kalra

Disclaimer

Auto-summaries can be generated by either an abstractive or extractive auto-summarization:

- An extraction-based summarizer identifies the most important sentences of a text and uses the original sentences to create the summary.
- An abstraction-based summarizer creates new text based on deep learning. New phrases are created to summarize the content.

The auto-summaries you will find in this book have been generated via an abstractive summarization approach.

Each chapter was carefully edited by Dr. Shilpa Chugh Garcha and Dr. Sanjay Kalra. The editors selected the papers which were then auto-summarized. The editors have edited the autosummaries to support the understanding of the original content. You will find the editors' reviews and guidance on the auto-summaries in their chapter introductions. In machine-generated books, editors are defined as those who curate the content for the book by selecting the papers to be auto-summarized and by organizing the output into a meaningful order. Next to the thoughtful curation of the papers, editors should guide the readers through the auto-summaries and make transparent why they selected the papers.

The ultimate goal is to provide a current literature review of Springer Nature publications on a given topic in order to support readers in overcoming information overload and to help them dive into a topic faster; to identify interdisciplinary overlaps; and to present papers that might not have been on the readers' radar.

Please note that the selected papers are not used to train an LLM while the auto-summaries are created.

Contents

About the Editors

Shilpa Chugh Garcha a pharmacologist, has a keen interest in the field of pharmaceutical research and development and healthcare education. With a postgraduation in Pharmacology (MBBS, MD), Dr. Shilpa worked as an Assistant Professor of Pharmacology at Shree Guru Gobind Singh Tricentenary (SGT) Medical College, Gurgaon, India, early in her career, followed by an opportunity to work as a medical affairs professional with pharmaceuticals like Novo Nordisk India and Baxter India. She also worked as a senior manager with the online healthcare organization https://www.1mg.com/ where she had the opportunity to work for patient education and other healthcare projects. Using her diverse work experience over the years, she is passionate about contributing to health education for patients and healthcare professionals.

Sanjay Kalra an endocrinologist at Bharti Hospital, Karnal, India, is a strong advocate of person-centered endocrinology, focusing on clinical care, education, and research. A Board member of the International Society of Endocrinology (ISE), he serves as its Treasurer, Education Working Group as well. As Past President of the Endocrine Society of India (ESI), and of the South Asian Federation of Endocrine Societies (SAFES), he has worked to build bonds and bridges among the global endocrine fraternity.

Currently Vice President, South Asian Obesity Forum, and President, Association for Longevity and Anti Aging medicine, the topics closest to his heart are motivational therapeutics and obesity management.

Dr. Sanjay serves on the editorial board of numerous national and international journals and textbooks, and has authored/edited 1200+ PubMed-indexed articles and chapters. As of July 2024, he has been cited over 26,000 times, leading to an H index of 72 and an i10-index of 458. He serves as Section Editor of the PubMed-indexed textbook, Endo Text, as well as Editor-in-Chief, Endocrine Society of India Textbook of Endocrinology. He rounds off his working days with his favorite hobbies, the traditional Indian folk dance, bhangra, and his exercise companion, the mugdar (Indian bell club).

Chapter 1
Introduction to Obesity and Anti-obesity Medications

Shilpa Chugh Garcha and Sanjay Kalra

According to the 2023 World Obesity Atlas report, 38% of the global population is either overweight or obese as of the year 2020, having a body mass index (BMI) higher than 25 kg/m^2, and is projected to reach 51% by 2035 [1].

This chapter includes studies on current trends in the prevalence of obesity worldwide, the economic implications of obesity, its management strategies, current pharmacotherapy options, and their targets. Some studies also discuss the history of the development of anti-obesity medications and the drugs which have been withdrawn over the years due to concerns over their adverse effects. In this chapter we have also discussed the drugs diethylpropion and phentermine that have been approved for short-term use in the management of obesity.

These studies highlight the increasing prevalence of obesity in low- and middle-income countries and how a plateau is emerging in high-income nations. The authors share their perspective on how obesity-related complications burden and influences the healthcare spending for people with obesity, their economic implications on nationwide healthcare costs, and the importance of preventive measures, early intervention, and effective weight management strategies.

A study included here engaged Italian experts in the field of obesity management to suggest a practical framework for clinicians and they advocated a shift of obesity management from BMI-focused guidelines to individualised treatment plans as per the risk profiles and associated health conditions. Many advances have occurred in the last decade in the management of obesity including lifestyle modifications, behavioural therapies, antiobesity pharmacotherapy, and bariatric surgery.

Lifestyle interventions play an important role in the management of obesity, however, there is difficulty in sustaining weight and there are high chances of weight

S. C. Garcha (✉)
Sonepat, Haryana, India

S. Kalra
Department of Endocrinology, Bharti Hospital, Karnal, Haryana, India

S. C. Garcha, S. Kalra (eds.), *Drugs for Medical Management of Obesity*,
https://doi.org/10.1007/978-981-96-1651-0_1

regain once the lifestyle interventions stop [2]. Bariatric surgery helps in sustained weight loss but is not accepted by many patients as it is invasive and carries the risk of long-term complications and peri-operative mortality. So, pharmacotherapy remains an important and essential intervention in the management of obesity [2].

An individual with a BMI of 25–29.9 kg/m^2 or $\geq$30 kg/m^2 is classified as being overweight or obese, however, with slight variations, a BMI of 23–24.9 kg/m^2 or $\geq$25 kg/m^2 in Asian populations is classified as overweight or obesity [3].

Antiobesity medications (AOMs) are indicated in people with a BMI higher than 30 kg/m^2, however, in people with a BMI more than 27 kg/m^2, AOMs are indicated if there are associated comorbidities. Obesity surgery is considered in people with a BMI higher than 40 kg/m^2 and in people with a BMI more than 35 kg/m^2 if there are associated comorbidities [4].

Various studies explore the central nervous system and other neuronal pathways that regulate appetite and body weight. The main area of focus has been the lateral hypothalamus, its role in influencing hedonic food behaviours and regulating food intake behaviours through brain reward areas along with the role of various neurotransmitters and neuropeptides, such as Agouti-related peptide and pro-opiomelanocortin neurons in the arcuate nucleus, which have shown opposing effects on food intake.

Studies included here discusses weight loss drugs including aminorex, fenfluramine, dexfenfluramine, phenylpropanolamine, sibutramine, rimonabant, and lorcaserin which have been withdrawn from the market over time due to their adverse event profiles. Serotonin and noradrenaline uptake inhibitor, sibutramine was withdrawn from the market due to its adverse effects on cardiovascular profile and cannabinoid type 1 receptor antagonist, rimonabant was withdrawn due to its adverse effects including depression and suicidal tendencies. Lorcaserin was initially not approved by the US Federal Drug Administration (USFDA) due to cancer risks in rats but was later approved based on clinical trials and was recently withdrawn when human trials revealed concerns over increased cancer risks.

Currently, two drugs Phentermine and Diethylpropion have been approved for short-term use only in the management of obesity by the US Federal Drug Administration USFDA. Drugs approved by USFDA for long-term weight loss include orlistat, an intestinal lipase inhibitor, fixed drug combinations that mainly act by appetite suppression (phentermine/topiramate and bupropion/naltrexone), GLP 1 receptor analogs (liraglutide 3.0 mg and semaglutide 2.4 mg), a novel *dual* GIP/GLP-1 receptor *agonist* (tirzepatide), and setmelanotide (for the treatment of a genetic disorder associated severe obesity).

This chapter includes studies on phentermine and diethylpropion, drugs approved by regulatory authorities for short-term use only. One study of phentermine discusses the addiction potential of phentermine on its long-term use and another explores its use in the management of pediatric obesity and its impact on weight, BMI, heart rate, and blood pressure and suggests further clinical studies to explore its long-term efficacy and safety. The study on diethylpropion explores its long-term effects on weight loss and its cardiovascular and psychiatric safety profile.

The studies highlight the need for anti-obesity medications with better efficacy and safety and to improve clinical outcomes that can significantly enhance the management of obesity with the help of multi-target agents and personalized therapeutic strategies. Drugs currently approved by USFDA are listed below (Table 1.1).

Table 1.1 USFDA approved anti-obesity medications

Drug name (Route)	USFDA approval (Year)	Age groups approved for	Mechanism of action
Short-term use (few weeks only)			
Phentermine (Oral) [5]	1959	Above 16 years	Sympathomimetic amine (anorectic)
Diethylpropion (Oral) [6]	1959	Above 16 years	Sympathomimetic amine
Long-term use			
Orlistat (Oral) [7]	1999 2007 (OTC use, Orlistat 60 mg)	12 years and above	Lipase inhibitor
Phentermine/ Topiramate (Oral) [8]	2012	12 years and above	Sympathomimetic amine/ GABA agonist, glutamate antagonist, carbonic anhydrase inhibitor
Naltrexone/ Bupropion (Oral) [9]	2014	18 years and above	Opioid antagonist/Dopamine and nor-adrenaline reuptake inhibitor
Liraglutide 3.0 (subcutaneous, once daily) [10]	2014	12 years and above and body weight >60 kg	Glucagon-like peptide-1 (GLP 1) receptor agonist
Semaglutide 2.4 (subcutaneous, once weekly) [11]	2021	12 years and above	Glucagon-like peptide-1 (GLP-1) receptor agonist
Tirzepatide (subcutaneous, once weekly) [12]	2023	18 years and above	Dual glucose-dependent insulinotropic polypeptide (GIP) receptor and glucagon-like peptide-1 (GLP-1) receptor agonist
Setmelanotide (subcutaneous, once daily) [13]	2020	6 years and above for monogenic syndromic obesity	Melanocortin 4 (MC4) receptor agonist
Metreleptin (subcutaneous) [14]	2014	Treatment of complications of leptin deficiency in patients with congenital or acquired generalized lipodystrophy	Activates the human leptin receptor (ObR)

References for Introduction

1. Lobstein T, Jackson-Leach R, Powis J, Brinsden H, Gray M. 2023. Available from: https://s3-eu-west-1.amazonaws.com/wof-files/World_Obesity_Atlas_2023_Report.pdf
2. Jones BJ, Bloom SR. The new era of drug therapy for obesity: the evidence and the expectations. Drugs 2015;75, 935–45. https://doi.org/10.1007/s40265-015-0410-1
3. BMI Classification for Obesity and overweight. https://iris.who.int/bitstream/handle/10665/206936/0957708211_eng.pdf
4. Apovian CM, Aronne LJ, Bessesen DH, McDonnell ME, Hassan Murad M, Pagotto U, Ryan DH, Still CD. Pharmacological management of obesity: an endocrine society clinical practice guideline. J Clin Endocrinol Metabol 2015;100(2):342–62. https://doi.org/10.1210/jc.2014-3415
5. Adipex-P (Phentermin). U.S. Food and Drug Administration website. https://www.accessdata.fda.gov/drugsatfda_docs/label/2012/085128s065lbl.pdf. Revised January 2012. Accessed Aug 6, 2024
6. Diethylproipion DailyMed - DIETHYLPROPION HYDROCHLORIDE tablet (nih.gov). Accessed in Sept 24
7. Xenical (Orlistat). U.S. Food and Drug Administration website. https://www.accessdata.fda.gov/drugsatfda_docs/label/2022/020766s038lbl.pdf. Revised August 2016. Accessed Aug 6, 2024
8. QSYMIA (phentermine and topiramate extended-release capsules). U.S. Food and Drug Administration website. https://www.accessdata.fda.gov/drugsatfda_docs/label/2023/022580s023lbl.pdf. Revised June 2024. Accessed Oct 19, 2024
9. CONTRAVE (naltrexone HCl and bupropion HCl) Extended Release Tablets. U.S. Food and Drug Administration website. https://www.accessdata.fda.gov/drugsatfda_docs/label/2014/200063s000lbl.pdf. Revised Sep 2014. Accessed Aug 8, 2024
10. SAXENDA (liraglutide) injection, U.S. Food and Drug Administration website. https://www.accessdata.fda.gov/drugsatfda_docs/label/2023/206321s016lbl.pdf. Revised Apr 2023. Accessed Aug 8, 2024
11. WEGOVY (semaglutide) injection. U.S. Food and Drug Administration website. https://www.accessdata.fda.gov/drugsatfda_docs/label/2023/215256s007lbl.pdf. Revised Jul 2023. Accessed Aug 8, 2024
12. ZEPBOUND® (tirzepatide) Injection. U.S. Food and Drug Administration website. https://www.accessdata.fda.gov/drugsatfda_docs/label/2024/217806s003lbl.pdf. Revised Mar 2024. Accessed Aug 8, 2024.
13. IMCIVREE® (setmelanotide) injection U.S. Food and Drug Administration website. https://www.accessdata.fda.gov/drugsatfda_docs/label/2022/213793s001lbl.pdf. Revised Jun 2022. Accessed Aug 8, 2024.
14. MYALEPT (metreleptin). U.S. Food and Drug Administration website. https://www.accessdata.fda.gov/drugsatfda_docs/label/2014/125390s004lbl.pdf. Revised Jun 2014. Accessed Aug 14, 2024

1.1 Machine Generated Summaries

Disclaimer: The summaries in this chapter were generated from Springer Nature publications using abstractive AI auto-summarization: An abstraction-based summarizer creates new text based on deep learning. New phrases are created to summarize the content. As the constituted sentences are machine selected, they may not fully reflect the body of the work, so we strongly advise that the original content is read and cited. The auto-generated summaries were curated by the editor to meet Springer Nature publication standards.

Machine generated keywords: phentermine, obesity prevalence, antiobesity drug, patient bmi.

Update on the Obesity Epidemic: After the Sudden Rise, Is the Upward Trajectory Beginning to Flatten? [153]

This is a machine-generated summary of:

Koliaki, Chrysi; Dalamaga, Maria; Liatis, Stavros: Update on the Obesity Epidemic: After the Sudden Rise, Is the Upward Trajectory Beginning to Flatten? [153]

Published in: Current Obesity Reports (2023)

Link to original: https://doi.org/10.1007/s13679-023-00527-y

If you want to cite the papers, please refer to the original.

For technical reasons we could not place the page where the original quote is coming from.

Research highlights

Introduction:

The global obesity epidemic, often termed "globesity," has become a critical public health issue, with the World Health Organization declaring it an epidemic. Obesity is associated with a range of chronic diseases and has significant morbidity and mortality. Despite some reports suggesting a stabilization of obesity rates in high-income countries, the overall trend continues to escalate, particularly in low- and middle-income populations. Now a new study by Chrysi Koliaki and colleagues provides an updated narrative review on current obesity prevalence trends, examining the evidence for a possible plateau in obesity rates and exploring the underlying factors contributing to the global obesity epidemic.

Main Body:

Koliaki et al. conducted a comprehensive literature search using databases such as PubMed, Medline, and Google Scholar to compile data on global and regional obesity trends from various sources including systematic reviews and epidemiological reports as per national databases. Their analysis reveals that while there has been a stabilization of obesity rates in some high-income countries post-2006, low- and middle-income countries continue to experience a sharp increase in prevalence. The study delves into the "energy balance flipping point hypothesis," which suggests that a critical switch occurred around 1960, leading to an exponential increase in 1980s. The access to energy-dense foods led to an increase in body weight and consequently an upward shift in energy expenditure requirements. The authors also discuss the "obesity transition" theory, which outlines four stages of obesity epidemiology based on economic progression and development in different countries.

Advances and Future Directions:

The main advance highlighted by Koliaki et al.'s review is the nuanced understanding of the complex dynamics driving the global obesity epidemic. While there is evidence for a plateau in some regions, particularly among children and adolescents in high-income countries, this stabilization is not universal. The authors emphasize that even if rates appear stable, they remain at alarmingly high levels with no guarantee against future increases. Koliaki et al. call for immediate effective actions at both population and regional levels to halt the escalating epidemic. They suggest that multi-component initiatives targeting both individual behavior and broader sociocultural determinants are urgently needed, backed by strong political will. As per the authors, the universal trend is obesity escalation rather than slowdown... it is imperative to intensify strategies targeting the epidemic. This research underscores the complexity of addressing globesity and points towards an integrated approach for future interventions.

Real-World Costs of Obesity-Related Complications over Eight Years: A US Retrospective Cohort Study in 28,500 Individuals [154]

This is a machine-generated summary of:

Pearson-Stuttard, Jonathan; Banerji, Tania; Capucci, Silvia; de Laguiche, Elisabeth; Faurby, Mads D.; Haase, Christiane Lundegaard; Sommer Matthiessen, Kasper; Near, Aimee M.; Tse, Jenny; Zhao, Xiaohui; Evans, Marc: Real-world costs of obesity-related complications over eight years: a US retrospective cohort study in 28,500 individuals [154]

Published in: International Journal of Obesity (2023)

Link to original: https://doi.org/10.1038/s41366-023-01376-4

Copyright of the summarized publication:

The Author(s) 2023

If you want to cite the papers, please refer to the original.

For technical reasons we could not place the page where the original quote is coming from.

Research highlights

Introduction:

The global obesity epidemic has reached alarming proportions, with a threefold increase in prevalence over the past four decades. In the United States, obesity rates are particularly high and continue to escalate, exacerbated by the COVID-19 pandemic. Obesity poses significant health risks, including cardiovascular diseases, dyslipidemia, type 2 diabetes, other metabolic complications, and osteoarthritis. These obesity related complications (ORCs) impose a substantial economic burden on healthcare systems. Despite previous research on the economic impact of ORCs, there remains a gap in understanding the long-term healthcare costs associated with ORCs on a national scale. Now a new study by Jonathan Pearson-Stuttard and colleagues addresses this gap by analyzing nationwide longitudinal data to assess the association between comorbidity burden and healthcare costs over time in individuals with obesity.

Main Body:

Pearson-Stuttard et al.'s retrospective cohort study utilized comprehensive databases, including the IQVIA Ambulatory Electronic Medical Records database with over 80 million patient records and PharMetrics Plus, encompassing over 210 million patient records. The study focused on adults with obesity, tracking their healthcare costs related to ORCs over several years. "Our analysis provides a unique perspective on how comorbidity burden influences healthcare spending in the obese population," explains Pearson-Stuttard. By employing sophisticated statistical models, the team adjusted for various factors such as age, sex, region, and obesity class to estimate annual costs for different ORC cohorts.

The study's robust methodology allowed for an accurate depiction of cost progression associated with ORCs in individuals with obesity. It revealed that direct healthcare costs were significantly higher for those with atleast one ORC compared to those without and that these costs escalated over time. The researchers also identified specific ORCs that drove these costs upward, providing valuable insights into which conditions might benefit from targeted preventative measures.

Conclusion:

Pearson-Stuttard's study marks a significant advance in our understanding of the economic implications of ORCs. "Our findings underscore the importance of early intervention and effective weight management strategies," Pearson-Stuttard asserts. By demonstrating that the number of ORCs is a more critical driver of healthcare costs than obesity severity alone, this research highlights the need for healthcare systems to prioritize managing and preventing ORCs to mitigate the financial strain of obesity. Looking ahead, these insights pave the way for future studies to explore comprehensive cost-saving approaches and inform policies aimed at reducing the long-term economic impact of obesity on society.

Updating Obesity Management Strategies: An Audit of Italian Specialists [155]

This is a machine-generated summary of:

Busetto, Luca; Carbonelli, Maria Grazia; Caretto, Antonio; Colao, Annamaria; Cricelli, Claudio; De Luca, Maurizio; Giorgino, Francesco; Gnessi, Lucio; Medea, Gerardo; Pappagallo, Giovanni; Santini, Ferruccio; Sbraccia, Paolo; Zappa, Marco Antonio: Updating obesity management strategies: an audit of Italian specialists [155]

Published in: Eating and Weight Disorders—Studies on Anorexia, Bulimia and Obesity (2022)

Link to original: https://doi.org/10.1007/s40519-022-01402-w

If you want to cite the papers, please refer to the original.

For technical reasons we could not place the page where the original quote is coming from.

Research highlights

Introduction:

Despite the global efforts to combat obesity, its prevalence continues to rise, posing significant health risks and economic burdens. The chronic low-grade inflammation, altered immune response to infections, and increased risk of comorbidities associated with obesity increases risk of hospitalization and mortality. However, current clinical guidelines often rely on body mass index (BMI) thresholds that may delay necessary interventions. Now a new study by Luca Busetto and colleagues addresses these shortcomings by proposing a more nuanced approach to obesity management that transcends BMI-centric models.

Main Body:

Busetto's team conducted a multicenter workshop using the Delphi method, engaging Italian experts in obesity management to reach a consensus on updating clinical practices. As per the authors, the aim was to provide a practical framework for clinicians, one that emphasizes early identification of risk factors and tailors treatment to individual patient needs. Over several months, the experts developed statements addressing key areas such as the limitations of BMI, the importance of additional anthropometric assessments, and the need for specific treatment targets.

The panelists rated their agreement with each statement using an online platform, achieving consensus on several key points. These included recognizing health conditions such as prediabetes as an indication for more aggressive therapy. For example, in patients with prediabetes considering anti-obesity medications if BMI is between 27–30 kg/m^2 and considering bariatric surgery in patients with BMI 35–40 kg/m^2 who cannot control their body weight with maximal medical therapy. The study's methodology ensured anonymity during surveys while facilitating open exchange during workshops, fostering a comprehensive and unbiased expert opinion.

Conclusion:

The study by Busetto et al. marks a significant advance in obesity management by advocating for a shift from BMI-focused guidelines to personalized care strategies. As per the authors, clinicians must consider the full psycho-physical complexity of patients. Looking ahead, this research paves the way for more effective interventions tailored to individual risk profiles and clinical conditions, potentially improving outcomes for people living with obesity.

Anti-obesity Drug Discovery: Advances and Challenges [156]

This is a machine-generated summary of:

Müller, Timo D.; Blüher, Matthias; Tschöp, Matthias H.; DiMarchi, Richard D.: Anti-obesity drug discovery: advances and challenges [156]

Published in: Nature Reviews Drug Discovery (2021)

Link to original: https://doi.org/10.1038/s41573-021-00337-8

If you want to cite the papers, please refer to the original.

For technical reasons we could not place the page where the original quote is coming from.

Research highlights

Introduction:

Control of excess body fat is a critical healthcare challenge, with obesity prevalence soaring globally and more than two-thirds of the US population affected by excess body weight. Obesity exacerbates numerous health conditions, including type 2 diabetes and various cancers, and has been a complicating factor in the COVID-19 pandemic. Despite the significant health risks and financial burdens associated with obesity, effective long-term treatment strategies remain elusive. Now a new study by Timo D. Müller and colleagues addresses this issue by reviewing the history of anti-obesity medications (AOMs), discussing ongoing challenges, and highlighting recent advances in AOM development.

Main Body:

Müller et al.'s comprehensive review delves into the complex interplay of genetic, environmental, and neuroendocrine factors contributing to obesity. The authors underscore the limitations of short-term behavioral interventions and the moderate efficacy of lifestyle changes, advocating for escalated treatment strategies that may include pharmacological interventions. They detail the journey from historical AOM failures including sibutramine, fenfluramine, dexfenfluramine, rainbow pills due to their adverse cardiovascular effects, rimonabant due to its increased suicidal risk and methamphetamine due to potential of drug dependence and abuse to recent breakthroughs such as FDA-approved liraglutide 3.0 mg and semaglutide 2.4 mg for chronic weight management. The study methodically examines the molecular mechanisms controlling appetite and energy utilization, emphasizing the translational value of rodent models in drug candidate selection. Müller et al. also explore endocrine control of food intake, discussing how various hormones act on the brain to regulate hunger and satiety.

Conclusion:

The main advances highlighted by Müller et al. include a better understanding of energy homeostasis mechanisms and the development of promising therapeutic candidates like semaglutide 2.4 mg. The authors suggest that future AOM strategies may involve targeting multiple mechanisms simultaneously to optimize disease management, drawing parallels with hypertension treatment approaches. Müller's quote encapsulates this vision: "It seems inevitable, and with good precedent, that such a conceptual approach to lowering body weight will eventually prevail." The study points towards an optimistic future for obesity pharmacotherapy, where drug-based management could potentially rival the efficacy of bariatric surgery.

Pharmacological Interventions for Obesity: Current and Future Targets [157]
This is a machine-generated summary of:

Bocarsly, Miriam E.: Pharmacological Interventions for Obesity: Current and Future Targets [157]

Published in: Current Addiction Reports (2018)

Link to original: https://doi.org/10.1007/s40429-018-0204-0

If you want to cite the papers, please refer to the original.

For technical reasons we could not place the page where the original quote is coming from.

Research highlights

Introduction:

Obesity in the United States has reached epidemic proportions, with a significant portion of the adult population classified as obese, leading to increased health risks and substantial economic costs. Despite extensive research into behavioral and lifestyle interventions, obesity rates have remained stubbornly high. Now a new study by Miriam E. Bocarsly delves into the neural mechanisms that govern energy intake and expenditure, offering insights into potential pharmacological interventions for obesity.

In their comprehensive review, Bocarsly explores the intricate network of brain regions and neuronal pathways that regulate appetite and body weight, with a particular focus on the hypothalamus. The author examines the role of various neurotransmitters and neuropeptides, such as Agouti-related peptide (AgRP) and pro-opiomelanocortin (POMC) neurons in the arcuate nucleus, which have opposing effects on food intake. The authors also discuss how hedonic or compulsive feeding factors influence eating behavior through brain reward systems like the lateral hypothalamus (LHA) and ventral tegmental area. By integrating findings from genetic tools and in vivo studies, they highlight how different neuronal populations within these regions contribute to feeding behaviors.

The review underscores the complexity of energy balance regulation and points to several promising pharmacological targets for obesity treatment. They suggest that future research should focus on understanding how exogenous compounds interact with central pathways to identify novel targets for drug development.

Conclusion:

The study by Miriam E. Bocarsly et al. represents a significant advance in our understanding of the central regulation of energy balance and its implications for obesity treatment. By elucidating the neural substrates involved in feeding behavior, this work paves the way for innovative pharmacological strategies targeting specific brain circuits. As Bocarsly notes, "Exploring targets relevant to addiction might lead to the way to new anti-obesity drugs," highlighting the potential crossover between addiction treatment and obesity management. The ultimate goal is to develop interventions that selectively curb hedonic overeating without affecting essential energy homeostasis, thereby addressing one of today's most pressing public health challenges.

The New Era of Drug Therapy for Obesity: The Evidence and the Expectations [158]

This is a machine-generated summary of:

Jones, Ben J.; Bloom, Stephen R.: The New Era of Drug Therapy for Obesity: The Evidence and the Expectations [158]

Published in: Drugs (2015)

Link to original: https://doi.org/10.1007/s40265-015-0410-1

If you want to cite the papers, please refer to the original.

For technical reasons we could not place the page where the original quote is coming from.

Research highlights

Introduction:

The global obesity epidemic is a growing concern, with millions of adults worldwide classified as obese, leading to increased risks of various diseases and healthcare challenges. Despite efforts to address environmental factors contributing to obesity, effective individual treatments are urgently needed. Now a new study by Ben J. Jones and Stephen R. Bloom delves into the physiology of energy homeostasis to identify pharmacological targets for weight reduction, assesses past and current treatments, and explores novel agents and regulatory challenges in managing obesity.

Main Body:

The authors provide a comprehensive review of the strategies for pharmacological weight loss by examining the mechanisms that govern energy balance—specifically, how various factors influence food intake and energy expenditure. The authors highlight the role of the hypothalamus in appetite regulation, where neurons respond to peripheral signals like glucose and hormones to modulate feeding behavior. They also discuss the potential of brown adipose tissue (BAT) activation for increasing energy expenditure, a relatively new area of research with therapeutic implications.

The study methodically reviews the history of anti-obesity pharmacotherapy, noting the safety concerns that have limited drug approvals in the past. It then transitions to an evaluation of current anti-obesity agents, detailing their mechanisms, efficacy, and side effects. The authors underscore the importance of pre-specified cardiovascular safety data for regulatory approval and emphasize that weight loss drugs are judged not only by their ability to reduce body weight but also by their impact on overall health outcomes.

Conclusion:

This review marks significant progress in obesity pharmacotherapy, with new treatments emerging after years of stagnation. The main advances include a better understanding of appetite regulation and energy homeostasis, leading to more targeted therapies. However, there remains a need for ongoing research into the safety profiles of these agents and their long-term effects. Looking forward, combination therapies targeting multiple pathways may offer more effective solutions for weight management. As Jones et al. suggest, "It remains to be seen whether medical therapy can achieve the robust weight loss of bariatric surgery," indicating a future direction for research that could potentially transform obesity treatment strategies.

Current Pharmacotherapy for Obesity [159]

This is a machine-generated summary of:

Srivastava, Gitanjali; Apovian, Caroline M.: Current pharmacotherapy for obesity [159]

Published in: Nature Reviews Endocrinology (2017)

Link to original: https://doi.org/10.1038/nrendo.2017.122

If you want to cite the papers, please refer to the original.

For technical reasons we could not place the page where the original quote is coming from.

Research highlights

Obesity has become a global epidemic, with its prevalence doubling in numerous countries and contributing to approximately four million deaths worldwide since 1981 due to its association with cardiovascular diseases and other comorbidities. In the United States, over one-third of adults are affected by obesity, which has seen a disproportionate rise in severity. Despite lifestyle interventions, many patients struggle to achieve and maintain weight loss, highlighting the need for effective pharmacological treatments. Now a new study by Gitanjali Srivastava and Caroline M. Apovian provides a timely review of current anti-obesity drugs, offering insights into their safety, efficacy, and clinical application, marking a step towards personalized obesity medicine.

This comprehensive review delves into the pharmacodynamics of FDA-approved anti-obesity medications such as phentermine, orlistat, phentermine/topiramate extended release (ER), lorcaserin, naltrexone sustained release (SR)/bupropion SR and liraglutide (the only injectable formulation). The authors detail the historical challenges of developing safe anti-obesity drugs due to past adverse effects but note that current medications primarily act on central nervous system pathways to reduce appetite or enhance satiety except orlistat that acts by inhibiting fat absorption. The review underscores the importance of understanding individual variations in response to these drugs, which is crucial for optimizing treatment efficacy. By examining clinical trials and real-world case studies, the authors provide a nuanced narrative on how these medications can be integrated into obesity management.

The study by Gitanjali Srivastava and Caroline M. Apovian represents a significant advance in the field of obesity treatment. It not only synthesizes current knowledge on anti-obesity pharmacotherapy but also points towards the future of personalized medicine in this domain. The authors suggest that identifying patient-specific obesity phenotypes could lead to more targeted and effective treatments. They advocate for continued research into pharmacometabonomics to predict individual responses to weight-loss medications. This research highlight underscores the potential for tailored therapeutic strategies that could revolutionize obesity care and improve patient outcomes significantly.

Long-term Efficacy and Safety of Anti-obesity Treatment: Where Do We Stand? [160]

This is a machine-generated summary of:

Tak, Young Jin; Lee, Sang Yeoup: Long-Term Efficacy and Safety of Anti-Obesity Treatment: Where Do We Stand? [160]

Published in: Current Obesity Reports (2021)

Link to original: https://doi.org/10.1007/s13679-020-00422-w

If you want to cite the papers, please refer to the original.

For technical reasons we could not place the page where the original quote is coming from.

Research highlights

Introduction:

Ischemic heart disease, cancer, and stroke, intricately linked to the obesity epidemic, remain the leading causes of death globally. The sedentary lifestyle and high-calorie diets prevalent in modern society, exacerbated by COVID-19 lockdowns, have fueled obesity rates. Now a new study by Young Jin Tak and Sang Yeoup Lee provides a comprehensive overview of the long-term efficacy and safety of anti-obesity drugs, offering insights into managing this complex chronic condition.

Main Body:

The authors meticulously reviewed the landscape of anti-obesity pharmacotherapy, emphasizing drugs withdrawn due to severe side effects such as aminorex, fenfluramine, dexfenfluramine, phenylpropanolamine, rimonabant, sibutramine, and lorcaserin. They detailed the mechanisms through which various medications operate, such as orlistat's inhibition of fat absorption, phentermine/topiramate and naltrexon/buropion's appetite suppression and slow gastric emptying and increased satiety by liraglutide. The study employed rigorous methods to evaluate the drugs' long-term impacts on weight management and associated health risks. For instance, lorcaserin's initial non-approval by the FDA due to cancer risks in rats followed by its approval basis the clinical trials conducted later was contrasted with its later market withdrawal after human trials revealed increased cancer incidence and non-approval of lorcaserin by European Medical Agency (EMA) due to potential risk of breast cancer, psychiatric adverse effects and valvulopathy as per its preclinical data. Similarly, orlistat's modest weight loss benefits were weighed against its gastrointestinal side effects and potential colorectal cancer risks.

Conclusion:

This review marks significant advances in understanding anti-obesity drugs' roles in long-term weight management. It points toward a future where tailored pharmacological interventions could complement lifestyle changes for individuals struggling with obesity. As one author notes, "The availability of different types of medications offers healthcare providers with more options to suggest tailored treatment plans for their patients." This research underscores the importance of safety in drug development and the need for ongoing surveillance post-approval. Looking ahead, it is clear that combating obesity will require a multifaceted approach that includes both lifestyle modifications and carefully managed pharmacotherapy.

Sibutramine and Rimonabant: A Postmortem Forensic Examination [161]

This is a machine-generated summary of:

Wittert, Gary: Sibutramine and Rimonabant: A Postmortem Forensic Examination [161]

Published in: (2013)

Link to original: https://doi.org/10.1007/978-1-4471-2834-2_28

If you want to cite the papers, please refer to the original.

For technical reasons we could not place the page where the original quote is coming from.

Research highlights

Obesity, a global health crisis, is often targeted through pharmacotherapy, with drugs like sibutramine and rimonabant once hailed as promising treatments due to their effects on satiety and metabolism. However, despite initial successes in weight loss, concerns have arisen regarding cardiovascular safety profiles of sibutramine and psychiatric adverse effects of rimonabant. Gary Wittert delves into the nuanced impacts of these drugs on cardio-metabolic risk factors and the reasons behind their market withdrawal.

Wittert conducted a comprehensive analysis, revealing that while sibutramine effectively lowers triglycerides and normalizes HDL cholesterol levels, it also consistently increases heart rate—a known risk factor for adverse cardiovascular outcomes. The Sibutramine Cardiovascular Outcomes (SCOUT) trial further highlighted an increased number of cardiovascular events among patients treated with sibutramine. Conversely, rimonabant showed potential in reducing blood pressure and triglycerides but was associated with significant psychiatric side effects, leading to its withdrawal from the market. The author explored data from clinical trials and real-world usage patterns, to assess the efficacy and safety of these anti-obesity medications.

While both drugs demonstrated weight loss benefits, their adverse effects on heart rate and mental health raised serious concerns. The author suggest that future drug development should be more cautious, prioritizing patient safety over rapid market introduction. They advocate for longer clinical trials that better reflect real-world populations and for regulatory bodies to require such comprehensive testing before approval. This analysis not only sheds light on the limitations of past treatments but also sets a precedent for more responsible drug development in addressing obesity and its comorbidities moving forward.

Addiction Potential of Phentermine Prescribed During Long-term Treatment of Obesity [162]

This is a machine-generated summary of:

Hendricks, E J; Srisurapanont, M; Schmidt, S L; Haggard, M; Souter, S; Mitchell, C L; De Marco, D G; Hendricks, M J; Istratiy, Y; Greenway, F L: Addiction potential of phentermine prescribed during long-term treatment of obesity [162]

Published in: International Journal of Obesity (2013)

Link to original: https://doi.org/10.1038/ijo.2013.74

If you want to cite the papers, please refer to the original.

For technical reasons we could not place the page where the original quote is coming from.

Research highlights

Introduction:

The global obesity crisis continues to escalate, with limited pharmacological interventions available to combat this health challenge. Despite the effectiveness of phentermine in short-term weight loss and long-term weight maintenance, concerns over its safety and potential for addiction have hindered its widespread use. Now a new study by E.J. Hendricks and colleagues addresses these concerns by investigating the addiction potential of phentermine in patients undergoing long-term treatment for obesity.

In this study, patients from a private obesity medicine specialty practice were recruited into two cohorts based on their duration of phentermine treatment—either long-term (minimum 1 year) or acute-term (7–14 days). The research utilized various psychometric scales, such as the Mini International Neuropsychiatric Interview (MINI-SUD), Cocaine Craving Questionnaire NOW (PCQ-NOW), and Amphetamine Withdrawal Questionnaire (PWQ), all modified for phentermine except Severity of Dependence Scale (SDS), to assess psychological dependence, abuse, craving, and amphetamine like withdrawal symptoms. The study's rigorous methodology included statistical analysis using ordinal data methods to ensure robust results.

The findings revealed no evidence of phentermine abuse or psychological dependence among long-term users. The SDS scores were low compared to known addictive substances, suggesting a minimal risk of addiction in a clinical setting.

Furthermore, craving assessments showed lower scores for long-term versus acute-term users, contradicting expectations if phentermine were truly addictive. Withdrawal symptoms were primarily characterized by increased appetite upon cessation rather than an amphetamine-like withdrawal symptom.

In conclusion, Hendricks et al.'s study provides compelling evidence that long-term phentermine use does not lead to addiction or induce drug craving and that concerns over potential addiction are likely overstated. This research paves the way for re-evaluating the role of phentermine in obesity treatment. As Hendricks notes, "These trial data suggest fears of causing addiction with long-term phentermine are exaggerated," which could significantly impact the future management of obesity worldwide.

Effect of Phentermine on Weight Reduction in a Pediatric Weight Management Clinic [163]

This is a machine-generated summary of:

Ryder, J R; Kaizer, A; Rudser, K D; Gross, A; Kelly, A S; Fox, C K: Effect of phentermine on weight reduction in a pediatric weight management clinic [163]

Published in: International Journal of Obesity (2016)

Link to original: https://doi.org/10.1038/ijo.2016.185

If you want to cite the papers, please refer to the original.

For technical reasons we could not place the page where the original quote is coming from.

Research highlights

Research Highlight

Obesity in youth presents a significant public health challenge, often necessitating pharmacotherapy alongside lifestyle modification to manage comorbid conditions or severe cases. Despite the widespread use of phentermine in adults, its efficacy and safety in pediatric obesity remain underexplored. Now a new study by J R Ryder and colleagues has conducted a retrospective chart review to assess the effectiveness of phentermine as an adjunct treatment to standard of care (SOC) lifestyle modification therapy in adolescents with obesity.

Ryder's team reviewed patient data from the University of Minnesota Masonic Children's Hospital Pediatric Weight Management Clinic, comparing those treated with phentermine plus SOC against a SOC-only group. The study meticulously matched the groups for baseline characteristics and employed generalized estimating equations to adjust for confounding factors. While the SOC included multidisciplinary support, the addition of phentermine was evaluated at several time points for its impact on weight, BMI, heart rate, and blood pressure. The researchers found that at 3 and 6 months, patients receiving phentermine plus SOC experienced significantly greater weight loss than those receiving SOC alone. Notably, heart rate increases (statistically significant at 3 months only) were observed in the phentermine group but without significant blood pressure changes.

The study marks an important step in pediatric obesity treatment, suggesting that phentermine could be a beneficial adjunct therapy. Future research should expand on these results through further clinical trials and explore long-term safety and efficacy, including impacts on cardiometabolic risk factors and quality of life. Ryder's work paves the way for more nuanced pharmacological strategies in combating pediatric obesity, potentially reshaping treatment paradigms for young populations at risk.

A Randomized Double-Blind Placebo-Controlled Study of the Long-term Efficacy and Safety of Diethylpropion in the Treatment of Obese Subjects [164]

This is a machine-generated summary of:

Cercato, C; Roizenblatt, V A; Leança, C C; Segal, A; Lopes Filho, A P; Mancini, M C; Halpern, A: A randomized double-blind placebo-controlled study of the long-term efficacy and safety of diethylpropion in the treatment of obese subjects [164]

Published in: International Journal of Obesity (2009)

Link to original: https://doi.org/10.1038/ijo.2009.124

If you want to cite the papers, please refer to the original.

For technical reasons we could not place the page where the original quote is coming from.

Research highlights

Introduction:

Obesity is a major health concern, increasing the risk of various chronic diseases and impacting overall mortality. Current long-term pharmacological interventions for obesity are limited, with sibutramine and orlistat being the only two drugs approved for extended use. Appetite-suppressant drugs offer a potential solution, yet their long-term efficacy and safety remain underexplored. Now a new study by Cercato and colleagues addresses this gap by evaluating the long-term effects of diethylpropion, an appetite suppressant with minor sympathomimetic properties, on weight loss and its cardiovascular and psychiatric safety profile.

Main Body:

Cercato's team conducted a rigorous randomized, double-blind, placebo-controlled trial at the Hospital das Clinicas, University of São Paulo-Brazil. The study spanned 6 months with an additional 6-month open-label extension. One hundred and one patients were recruited, adhering to strict inclusion criteria to minimize confounding variables. Participants were randomized to receive either diethylpropion or placebo while following a hypocaloric diet and increasing physical activity levels and were counselled to do atleast 150 min of physical activity per week.

The researchers meticulously monitored medication compliance, adverse events, and changes in weight, waist circumference, blood pressure, and metabolic parameters such as serum glucose, insulin, and lipids throughout the study duration.

The results revealed that diethylpropion led to significant weight loss compared to placebo over the initial 6 months. Furthermore, during the open-label extension where all participants received diethylpropion, continued weight reduction was observed. Importantly, no significant differences in cardiovascular risk factors were found between the treatment groups except for triglyceride levels. Adverse events were mild to moderate and decreased over time.

Conclusion:

The study by Cercato et al. marks a significant advance in understanding the long-term use of diethylpropion for obesity treatment. The authors report that diethylpropion not only effectively promotes weight loss but also positively influences cardiometabolic risk factors without severe adverse cardiovascular or psychiatric effects in a carefully selected patient population. However, they caution that their results are based on a predominantly female sample from a single center and may not be generalizable across genders or broader populations.

Bibliography

1. Mitchell RT, McDougall CM, Crum JE. Decreasing prevalence of obesity in primary schoolchildren. Arch Dis Child. 2007;92:153–4.
2. Tambalis KD, Panagiotakos DB, Kavouras SA, Kallistratos AA, Moraiti IP, Douvis SJ, et al. Eleven-year prevalence trends of obesity in Greek children: first evidence that prevalence of obesity is leveling off. Obesity. 2010;18:161–6.
3. Olds TS, Harten NR. One hundred years of growth: the evolution of height, mass, and body composition in Australian children, 1899–1999. Hum Biol. 2001;73:727–38.
4. Ogden CL, Carroll MD, Flegal KM. High body mass index for age among US children and adolescents, 2003–2006. JAMA. 2008;299:2401–5.
5. Lissner L, Sohlström A, Sundblom E, Sjöberg A. Trends in overweight and obesity in Swedish schoolchildren 1999–2005: has the epidemic reached a plateau?: national prevalence of obesity. Obes Rev. 2010:553–9.
6. Keane E, Kearney PM, Perry IJ, Kelleher CC, Harrington JM. Trends and prevalence of overweight and obesity in primary school aged children in the Republic of Ireland from 2002–2012: a systematic review. BMC Public Health. 2014;14
7. Wijnhoven TM, Van Raaij JM, Spinelli A, Starc G, Hassapidou M, Spiroski I, et al. WHO European childhood obesity surveillance initiative: body mass index and level of overweight among 6–9-year-old children from school year 2007/2008 to school year 2009/2010. BMC Public Health. 2014;14
8. Touloumi G, Karakosta A, Kalpourtzi N, Gavana M, Vantarakis A, Kantzanou M, et al. High prevalence of cardiovascular risk factors in adults living in Greece: the EMENO National Health Examination Survey. BMC Public Health. 2020;20:1665. This paper presents national data on the prevalence of cardiovascular risk factors, including obesity, in Greek adults between 2013 and 2016, based on the findings of the national health examination survey EMENO. According to these data, the prevalence of obesity in the Greek adult population is alarmingly high
9. Siopis G, Moschonis G, Reppas K, Iotova V, Bazdarska Y, Chakurova N, et al. The emerging prevalence of obesity within families in Europe and its associations with family sociodemographic characteristics and lifestyle factors; a cross-sectional analysis of baseline data from the Feel4Diabetes Study. Nutrients. 2023;15:1283. This cross-sectional analysis of baseline data from the Feel4Diabetes Study, reported high obesity prevalence rates in Greek

children of school age and examined the associations of obesity with sociodemographic and lifestyle characteristics of the affected families, emphasizing the need for tailored, family-based, interventions for obesity prevention
10. Lobstein T, Jackson-Leach R, Powis J, Brinsden H, Gray M. 2023. Available from: https://www.worldobesity.org/resources/resource-library/world-obesity-atlas-2023. Compiled by the World Obesity Federation, the World Obesity Atlas 2023 provides obesity prevalence projections and insights into the growing economic impact of overweight/obesity for the period 2020–2035. Alarmingly, over half of the global population is expected to have a high body mass index by the end of this period, and 1 in 4 people will be living with obesity compared to 1 in 7 today. Childhood obesity rates are rising very fast, and lower income countries are facing rapid increases in obesity prevalence.
11. Di Cesare M, Bentham J, Stevens GA, Zhou B, Danaei G, Lu Y, et al. Trends in adult body-mass index in 200 countries from 1975 to 2014: a pooled analysis of 1698 population-based measurement studies with 19.2 million participants. Lancet. 2016;387:1377–96.
12. Ng M, Fleming T, Robinson M, Thomson B, Graetz N, Margono C, et al. Global, regional, and national prevalence of overweight and obesity in children and adults during 1980–2013: a systematic analysis for the Global Burden of Disease Study 2013. Lancet. 2014;384:766–81.
13. Finucane MM, Stevens GA, Cowan MJ, Danaei G, Lin JK, Paciorek CJ, et al. National, regional, and global trends in body-mass index since 1980: systematic analysis of health examination surveys and epidemiological studies with 960 country-years and 9·1 million participants. Lancet. 2011;377:557–67.
14. Rokholm B, Baker JL, Sørensen TIA. The levelling off of the obesity epidemic since the year 1999-a review of evidence and perspectives. Obes Rev. 2010:835–46.
15. Staub K, Bender N, Floris J, Pfister C, Rühli FJ. From undernutrition to overnutrition: the evolution of overweight and obesity among young men in Switzerland since the 19th century. Obes Facts. 2016;9:259–72.
16. Drewnowski A, Popkin BM. The nutrition transition: new trends in the global diet. Nutr Rev. 1997;55:31–43.
17. Astrup A, Brand-Miller J. Diet composition and obesity. Lancet. 2012;379:1100; author reply 1100–1
18. Prentice A, Jebb S. Energy intake/physical activity interactions in the homeostasis of body weight regulation. Nutr Rev. 2004;62:S98–104.
19. Popkin BM, Adair LS, Ng SW. Global nutrition transition and the pandemic of obesity in developing countries. Nutr Rev. 2012;70:3–21.
20. Church TS, Thomas DM, Tudor-Locke C, Katzmarzyk PT, Earnest CP, Rodarte RQ, et al. Trends over 5 decades in U.S. occupation-related physical activity and their associations with obesity. PLoS One. 2011:6.
21. Swinburn B, Sacks G, Ravussin E. Increased food energy supply is more than sufficient to explain the US epidemic of obesity. Am J Clin Nutr. 2009;90:1453–6.
22. Scarborough P, Burg MR, Foster C, Swinburn B, Sacks G, Rayner M, et al. Increased energy intake entirely accounts for increase in body weight in women but not in men in the UK between 1986 and 2000. Br J Nutr. 2011;105:1399–404.
23. Jaacks LM, Vandevijvere S, Pan A, CJ MG, Wallace C, Imamura F, et al. The obesity transition: stages of the global epidemic. Lancet Diabetes Endocrinol. 2019;7:231–40. This paper described the evolving stages of obesity epidemiology in countries of different economic development by means of a four-stage conceptual model, the so-called "obesity transition model". This model is intended to provide guidance to policy makers in identifying the current stage of the obesity transition in a population, and implementing preventive measures to attenuate the transition, taking into account local contextual factors
24. Wang Y, Beydoun MA, Min J, Xue H, Kaminsky LA, Cheskin LJ. Has the prevalence of overweight, obesity and central obesity levelled off in the United States? Trends, patterns, disparities, and future projections for the obesity epidemic. Int J Epidemiol. 2021;49:810–23. Based on large national databases, this analysis examined time trends in obesity prevalence

across different socio-economic strata and geographic regions and made projections for the future course of the obesity epidemic in the USA. It was shown that obesity prevalence has been steadily rising since 1999, both in US adults and children/adolescents, despite some temporary stabilization (plateau) phases. There were great disparities across socioeconomic groups and geographical regions. The paper emphasized the need for effective, sustainable and culturally-tailored interventions

25. Benson L, Baer HJ, Kaelber DC. Trends in the diagnosis of overweight and obesity in children and adolescents: 1999–2007. Pediatrics. 2009;123:e153–8.
26. Olds TS, Tomkinson GR, Ferrar KE, Maher CA. Trends in the prevalence of childhood overweight and obesity in Australia between 1985 and 2008. Int J Obes. 2010;34:57–66.
27. Stamatakis E, Zaninotto P, Falaschetti E, Mindell J, Head J. Time trends in childhood and adolescent obesity in England from 1995 to 2007 and projections of prevalence to 2015. J Epidemiol Community Health. 1978;2010(64):167–74.
28. Sjöberg A, Lissner L, Albertsson-Wikland K, Mårild S. Recent anthropometric trends among Swedish school children: evidence for decreasing prevalence of overweight in girls. Acta Paediatr. 2008;97:118–23.
29. Romon M, Lommez A, Tafflet M, Basdevant A, Oppert JM, Bresson JL, et al. Downward trends in the prevalence of childhood overweight in the setting of 12-year school- and community-based programmes. Public Health Nutr. 2009;12:1735–42.
30. Péneau S, Salanave B, Maillard-Teyssier L, Rolland-Cachera M-F, Vergnaud A-C, Méjean C, et al. Prevalence of overweight in 6- to 15-year-old children in central/western France from 1996 to 2006: trends toward stabilization. Int J Obes. 2009;33:401–7.
31. Pearson S, Hansen B, Sørensen TIA, Baker JL. Overweight and obesity trends in Copenhagen schoolchildren from 2002 to 2007. Acta Paediatr. 2010;99:1675–8.
32. Kolle E, Steene-Johannessen J, Holme I, Andersen LB, Anderssen SA. Secular trends in adiposity in Norwegian 9-year-olds from 1999–2000 to 2005. BMC Public Health. 2009;9:389.
33. de Wilde JA, van Dommelen P, Middelkoop BJC, Verkerk PH. Trends in overweight and obesity prevalence in Dutch, Turkish, Moroccan and Surinamese South Asian children in The Netherlands. Arch Dis Child. 2009;94:795–800.
34. Stamatakis E, Wardle J, Cole TJ. Childhood obesity and overweight prevalence trends in England: evidence for growing socioeconomic disparities. Int J Obes. 2010;34:41–7.
35. Bergström E, Blomquist HKS. Is the prevalence of overweight and obesity declining among 4-year-old Swedish children? Acta Paediatr. 2009;98:1956–8.
36. Schmidt Morgen C, Rokholm B, Sjöberg Brixval C, Schou Andersen C, Geisler Andersen L, Rasmussen M, et al. Trends in prevalence of overweight and obesity in danish infants, children and adolescents–are we still on a plateau? PLoS One. 2013;8:e69860.
37. Abarca-Gómez L, Abdeen ZA, Hamid ZA, Abu-Rmeileh NM, Acosta-Cazares B, Acuin C, et al. Worldwide trends in body-mass index, underweight, overweight, and obesity from 1975 to 2016: a pooled analysis of 2416 population-based measurement studies in 128·9 million children, adolescents, and adults. Lancet [Internet]. 2017;390:2627–42. Available from: https://linkinghub.elsevier.com/retrieve/pii/S0140673617321293
38. Grammatikopoulou MG, Poulimeneas D, Gounitsioti IS, Gerothanasi K, Tsigga M, Kiranas E. Prevalence of simple and abdominal obesity in Greek adolescents: the ADONUT study. Clin Obes [Internet]. 2014; Available from: https://onlinelibrary.wiley.com/doi/10.1111/cob.12070
39. Walls HL, Peeters A, Proietto J, McNeil JJ. Public health campaigns and obesity-a critique. BMC Public Health. 2011;11:136.
40. Iannotti RJ, Wang J. Trends in physical activity, sedentary behavior, diet, and BMI among US adolescents, 2001–2009. Pediatrics. 2013;132:606–14.
41. Uro-Chukwu H, Liu X, Malakan Rad E, Zeng Z, Hu B, Li Q. The global burden of type 2 diabetes attributable to high body mass index in 204 countries and territories, 1990–2019: an analysis of the Global Burden of Disease Study.

42. Yang C, Jia X, Wang Y, Fan J, Zhao C, Yang Y, et al. Trends and influence factors in the prevalence, intervention, and control of metabolic syndrome among US adults, 1999–2018. BMC Geriatr. 2022;22
43. Younossi ZM, Golabi P, Paik JM, Henry A, Van Dongen C, Henry L. The global epidemiology of nonalcoholic fatty liver disease (NAFLD) and nonalcoholic steatohepatitis (NASH): a systematic review. Hepatology. 2023;77:1335–47.
44. Wang D, Xu Y, Zhu Z, Li Y, Li X, Li Y, et al. Changes in the global, regional, and national burdens of NAFLD from 1990 to 2019: a systematic analysis of the global burden of disease study 2019. Front Nutr. 2022:9.
45. Colditz GA, Peterson LL. Obesity and cancer: evidence, impact, and future directions. Clin Chem. 2018;64:154–62.
46. Li Q, Blume SW, Huang JC, Hammer M, Ganz ML. Prevalence and healthcare costs of obesity-related comorbidities: evidence from an electronic medical records system in the United States. J Med Econ. 2015;18:1020–8.
47. Divino V, Ramasamy A, Anupindi VR, Eriksen KT, Olsen AH, DeKoven M, et al. Complication-specific direct medical costs by body mass index for 13 obesity-related complications: a retrospective database study. J Manag Care Spec Pharm. 2021;27:210–22.
48. Padula WV, Allen RR, Nair KV. Determining the cost of obesity and its common comorbidities from a commercial claims database. Clin Obes. 2014;4:53–8.
49. Yumuk V, Tsigos C, Fried M, Schindler K, Busetto L, Micic D, Toplak H, Obesity Management Task Force of the European Association for the Study of Obesity. European guidelines for obesity management in adults. Obes Facts. 2015;8:402–24. https://doi.org/10.1159/000442721.
50. Rowe G, Wright G. Expert opinions in forecasting: role of the Delphi technique. In: Armstrong JS, editor. Principles of forecasting. Norwell: Kluwer Academic Press; 2001.
51. Busetto L, Sbraccia P, Vettor R. Obesity management: at the forefront against disease stigma and therapeutic inertia. Eat Weight Disord. 2021; https://doi.org/10.1007/s40519-021-01217-1.
52. Muller TD, Finan B, Clemmensen C, DiMarchi RD, Tschop MH. The new biology and pharmacology of glucagon. Physiol Rev. 2017;97:721–66.
53. Carlsson LMS, et al. Life expectancy after bariatric surgery in the Swedish Obese Subjects Study. N Engl J Med. 2020;383:1535–43.
54. Wilding JPH, et al. Once-weekly semaglutide in adults with overweight or obesity. N Engl J Med. 2021:384–989. This article shows the metabolic effects of semaglutide 2.4 mg in patients with obesity without diabetes
55. Nissen SE, et al. Effect of naltrexone–bupropion on major adverse cardiovascular events in overweight and obese patients with cardiovascular risk factors: a randomized clinical trial. JAMA. 2016;315:990–1004.
56. Dostalova I, Haluzikova D, Haluzik M. Fibroblast growth factor 21: a novel metabolic regulator with potential therapeutic properties in obesity/type 2 diabetes mellitus. Physiol Res. 2009;58:1–7.
57. Talukdar S, et al. A long-acting FGF21 molecule, PF-05231023, decreases body weight and improves lipid profile in non-human primates and type 2 diabetic subjects. Cell Metab. 2016;23:427–40.
58. Afshin A, et al. Health effects of overweight and obesity in 195 countries over 25 years. N Engl J Med. 2017;377:13–27. This article summarizes the prevalence rates and health consequences of obesity from 1990 until 2015
59. Global, B. M. I. M. C, et al. Body-mass index and all-cause mortality: individual-participant-data meta-analysis of 239 prospective studies in four continents. Lancet. 2016;388:776–86.
60. Twig G, et al. Body-mass index in 2.3 million adolescents and cardiovascular death in adulthood. N Engl J Med. 2016;374:2430–40.
61. Kleinert M, et al. Animal models of obesity and diabetes mellitus. Nat Rev Endocrinol. 2018;14:140–62.

62. Pi-Sunyer X, et al. A randomized, controlled trial of 3.0 mg of liraglutide in weight management. N Engl J Med. 2015;373:11–22.
63. Marso SP, et al. Liraglutide and cardiovascular outcomes in type 2 diabetes. N Engl J Med. 2016;375:311–22. This article shows the beneficial effects of liraglutide on cardiovascular health
64. Marso SP, et al. Effects of liraglutide on cardiovascular outcomes in patients with diabetes with or without heart failure. J Am Coll Cardiol. 2020;75:1128–41.
65. Frias JP, et al. Efficacy and tolerability of tirzepatide, a dual glucose-dependent insulinotropic peptide and glucagon-like peptide-1 receptor agonist in patients with type 2 diabetes: a 12-week, randomized, double-blind, placebo-controlled study to evaluate different dose-escalation regimens. Diabetes Obes Metab. 2020;22:938–46.
66. Fryar CD, Carroll MD, Ogden CL. Prevalence of overweight, obesity, and extreme obesity among adults aged 20 and over: United States, 1960–1962 through 2013–2014; 2016.
67. Flegal KM, Kruszon-Moran D, Carroll MD, Fryar CD, Ogden CL. Trends in obesity among adults in the United States, 2005 to 2014. JAMA. 2016;315:2284–91.
68. Fan W, Boston BA, Kesterson RA, Hruby VJ, Cone RD. Role of melanocortinergic neurons in feeding and the agouti obesity syndrome. Nature. 1997;385:165–8.
69. Jennings JH, Ung RL, Resendez SL, et al. Visualizing hypothalamic network dynamics for appetitive and consummatory behaviors. Cell. 2015;160:516–27. While it has been long indicated that the lateral hypothalamus is involved in feeding behaviors, this paper elegantly begins to tease apart the specific contributions of different cell types within the brain region
70. Qualls-Creekmore E, Yu S, Francois M, Hoang J, Huesing C, Bruce-Keller A, et al. Galanin-expressing GABA neurons in the lateral hypothalamus modulate food reward and noncompulsive locomotion. J Neurosci. 2017;37:6053–65.
71. Inutsuka A, Inui A, Tabuchi S, Tsunematsu T, Lazarus M, Yamanaka A. Concurrent and robust regulation of feeding behaviors and metabolism by orexin neurons. Neuropharmacology. 2014;85:451–60.
72. Haynes AC, Chapman H, Taylor C, Moore GBT, Cawthorne MA, Tadayyon M, et al. Anorectic, thermogenic and anti-obesity activity of a selective orexin-1 receptor antagonist in ob/ob mice. Regul Pept. 2002;104:153–9.
73. Kojima M, Kangawa K. Ghrelin: structure and function. Physiol Rev. 2005;85:495–522.
74. Dickson SL, Egecioglu E, Landgren S, Skibicka KP, Engel JA, Jerlhag E. The role of the central ghrelin system in reward from food and chemical drugs. Mol Cell Endocrinol. 2011;340:80–7.
75. Velazquez A, Apovian CM. Updates on obesity pharmacotherapy. Ann N Y Acad Sci. 2018;1411:106–19.
76. Bray GA, Frühbeck G, Ryan DH, Wilding JPH. Management of obesity. Lancet. 2016;387:1947–56.
77. Apovian CM, Istfan NW. Obesity: guidelines, best practices, new research. Endocrinol Metab Clin N Am. 2016;45:xvii–xviii.
78. McElroy SL, Hudson JI, Mitchell JE, Wilfley D, Ferreira-Cornwell MC, Gao J, et al. Efficacy and safety of lisdexamfetamine for treatment of adults with moderate to severe binge-eating disorder: a randomized clinical trial. JAMA Psychiatry. 2015;72:235–46.
79. Kakkar AK, Dahiya N. Drug treatment of obesity: current status and future prospects. Eur J Intern Med. 2015;26:89–94.
80. Hendricks EJ. Off-label drugs for weight management. Diabetes, Metab Syndr Obes Targets Ther. 2017;10:223–34.
81. Ahima RS, Antwi DA. Brain regulation of appetite and satiety. Endocrinol Metab Clin N Am. 2008;37:811–23.
82. World Health Organization. Global status report on noncommunicable diseases 2014 [Internet]. apps.who.int. [cited 2015 Mar 1]. Available from: http://apps.who.int/iris/bitstream/10665/148114/1/9789241564854_eng.pdf?ua=1.

83. Kelly T, Yang W, Chen C-S, Reynolds K, He J. Global burden of obesity in 2005 and projections to 2030. Int J Obes. 2008;32(9):1431–7.
84. Suzuki K, Simpson KA, Minnion JS, Shillito JC, Bloom SR. The role of gut hormones and the hypothalamus in appetite regulation. Endocr J. 2010;57(5):359–72.
85. Poher A-L, Altirriba J, Veyrat-Durebex C, Rohner-Jeanrenaud F. Brown adipose tissue activity as a target for the treatment of obesity/insulin resistance. Front Physiol. 2015;6:4.
86. Billington CJ, Briggs JE, Grace M, Levine AS. Effects of intracerebroventricular injection of neuropeptide Y on energy metabolism. Am J Phys. 1991;260(2 Pt 2):R321–7.
87. Morgan DA, McDaniel LN, Yin T, Khan M, Jiang J, Acevedo MR, et al. Regulation of glucose tolerance and sympathetic activity by MC4R signaling in the lateral hypothalamus. Diabetes. 2015; https://doi.org/10.2337/db14-1257.
88. Caricilli AM, Penteado E, de Abreu LL, Quaresma PGF, Santos AC, Guadagnini D, et al. Topiramate treatment improves hypothalamic insulin and leptin signaling and action and reduces obesity in mice. Endocrinology. 2012;153(9):4401–11.
89. Beiroa D, Imbernon M, Gallego R, Senra A, Herranz D, Villarroya F, et al. GLP-1 agonism stimulates brown adipose tissue thermogenesis and browning through hypothalamic AMPK. Diabetes. 2014;63(10):3346–58.
90. Goldstein DJ. Beneficial health effects of modest weight loss. Int J Obes Relat Metab Disord. 1992;16(6):397–415.
91. Knowler WC, Barrett-Connor E, Fowler SE, Hamman RF, Lachin JM, Walker EA, et al. Reduction in the incidence of type 2 diabetes with lifestyle intervention or metformin. N Engl J Med. 2002;346(6):393–403.
92. Look AHEAD Research Group. Effect of a long-term behavioural weight loss intervention on nephropathy in overweight or obese adults with type 2 diabetes: a secondary analysis of the Look AHEAD randomised clinical trial. Lancet Diabetes Endocrinol. 2014;2(10):801–9.
93. Christensen R, Bartels EM, Astrup A, Bliddal H. Effect of weight reduction in obese patients diagnosed with knee osteoarthritis: a systematic review and meta-analysis. Ann Rheum Dis. 2007;66(4):433–9.
94. James WPT, Caterson ID, Coutinho W, Finer N, Van Gaal LF, Maggioni AP, et al. Effect of sibutramine on cardiovascular outcomes in overweight and obese subjects. N Engl J Med. 2010;363(10):905–17.
95. Topol EJ, Bousser M-G, Fox KAA, Creager MA, Despres J-P, Easton JD, et al. Rimonabant for prevention of cardiovascular events (CRESCENDO): a randomised, multicentre, placebo-controlled trial. Lancet. 2010;376(9740):517–23.
96. Ben-Menachem E, Henriksen O, Dam M, Mikkelsen M, Schmidt D, Reid S, et al. Double-blind, placebo-controlled trial of topiramate as add-on therapy in patients with refractory partial seizures. Epilepsia. 1996;37(6):539–43.
97. Allison DB, Gadde KM, Garvey WT, Peterson CA, Schwiers ML, Najarian T, et al. Controlled-release phentermine/topiramate in severely obese adults: a randomized controlled trial (EQUIP). Obesity. 2012;20:330–42.
98. Wadden TA, Foreyt JP, Foster GD, Hill JO, Klein S, O'Neil PM, et al. Weight loss with naltrexone SR/bupropion SR combination therapy as an adjunct to behavior modification: the COR-BMOD trial. Obesity (Silver Spring). 2011;19(1):110–20.
99. Greenway FL, Fujioka K, Plodkowski RA, Mudaliar S, Guttadauria M, Erickson J, et al. Effect of naltrexone plus bupropion on weight loss in overweight and obese adults (COR-I): a multicentre, randomised, double-blind, placebo-controlled, phase 3 trial. Lancet. 2010;376:595–605.
100. Nahmias C, Blin N, Elalouf JM, Mattei MG, Strosberg AD, Emorine LJ. Molecular characterization of the mouse beta 3-adrenergic receptor: relationship with the atypical receptor of adipocytes. EMBO J. 1991;10(12):3721–7.
101. Berkowitz DE, Nardone NA, Smiley RM, Price DT, Kreutter DK, Fremeau RT, et al. Distribution of beta 3-adrenoceptor mRNA in human tissues. Eur J Pharmacol. 1995;289(2):223–8.

102. Fujimura T, Tamura K, Tsutsumi T, Yamamoto T, Nakamura K, Koibuchi Y, et al. Expression and possible functional role of the beta3-adrenoceptor in human and rat detrusor muscle. J Urol. 1999;161(2):680–5.
103. Batterham RL, Cowley MA, Small CJ, Herzog H, Cohen MA, Dakin CL, et al. Gut hormone PYY(3–36) physiologically inhibits food intake. Nature. 2002;418(6898):650–4.
104. Miras AD, le Roux CW. Can medical therapy mimic the clinical efficacy or physiological effects of bariatric surgery? Int J Obes. 2014;38(3):325–33.
105. Finan B, Yang B, Ottaway N, Smiley DL, Ma T, Clemmensen C, et al. A rationally designed monomeric peptide triagonist corrects obesity and diabetes in rodents. Nat Med. 2015;21(1):27–36.
106. Gloy VL, Briel M, Bhatt DL, Kashyap SR, Schauer PR, Mingrone G, et al. Bariatric surgery versus non-surgical treatment for obesity: a systematic review and meta-analysis of randomised controlled trials. BMJ. 2013;347:f5934.
107. Apovian CM, Aronne LJ, Bessesen DH, McDonnell ME, Murad MH, Pagotto U, et al. Pharmacological management of obesity: an endocrine society clinical practice guideline. J Clin Endocrinol Metab. 2015;100:342–62.
108. Zheng H, Lenard NR, Shin AC, Berthoud HR. Appetite control and energy balance regulation in the modern world: reward-driven brain overrides repletion signals. Int J Obes. 2009;33(Suppl. 2):S8–S13.
109. Lenard NR, Berthoud HR. Central and peripheral regulation of food intake and physical activity: pathways and genes. Obesity (Silver Spring). 2008;16(Suppl. 3):S11–22.
110. Berthoud HR. Interactions between the "cognitive" and "metabolic" brain in the control of food intake. Physiol Behav. 2007;91:486–98.
111. Bhasin S, Wallace W, Lawrence JB, Lesch M. Sudden death associated with thyroid hormone abuse. Am J Med. 1981;71:887–90.
112. Weintraub M, Sundaresan PR, Madan M, Schuster B, Balder A, Lasagna L, et al. Long-term weight control study. I (weeks 0 to 34). The enhancement of behavior modification, caloric restriction, and exercise by fenfluramine plus phentermine versus placebo. Clin Pharmacol Ther. 1992;51(5):586–94.
113. Weintraub M. Long-term weight control study: conclusions. Clin Pharmacol Ther. 1992;51:642–6.
114. Caterson ID, et al. Maintained intentional weight loss reduces cardiovascular outcomes: results from the Sibutramine cardiovascular OUTcomes (SCOUT) trial. Diabetes Obes Metab. 2012;14:523–30.
115. Munro JF, MacCuish AC, Wilson EM, Duncan LJ. Comparison of continuous and intermittent anorectic therapy in obesity. Br Med J. 1968;1:352–4.
116. Aronne LJ, Wadden TA, Peterson C, Winslow D, Odeh S, Gadde KM. Evaluation of phentermine and topiramate versus phentermine/topiramate extended-release in obese adults. Obesity. 2013;21:2163–71.
117. Torgerson JS, Hauptman J, Boldrin MN, Sjöström L. XENical in the prevention of diabetes in obese subjects (XENDOS) study: a randomized study of orlistat as an adjunct to lifestyle changes for the prevention of type 2 diabetes in obese patients. Diabetes Care. 2004;27:155–61.
118. Heymsfield SB, et al. Effects of weight loss with orlistat on glucose tolerance and progression to type 2 diabetes in obese adults. Arch Intern Med. 2000;160:1321–6.
119. Derosa G, Mugellini A, Ciccarelli L, Fogari R. Randomized, double-blind, placebo-controlled comparison of the action of orlistat, fluvastatin, or both an anthropometric measurements, blood pressure, and lipid profile in obese patients with hypercholesterolemia prescribed a standardized diet. Clin Ther. 2003;25:1107–22.
120. Gadde KM, Allison DB, Ryan DH, Peterson CA, Troupin B, Schwiers ML, et al. Effects of low-dose, controlled-release, phentermine plus topiramate combination on weight and associated comorbidities in overweight and obese adults (CONQUER): a randomised, placebo-controlled, phase 3 trial. Lancet. 2011;377:1341–52.

121. Garvey WT, Ryan DH, Look M, Gadde KM, Allison DB, Peterson CA, Schwiers M, Day WW, Bowden CH. Two-year sustained weight loss and metabolic benefits with controlled-release phentermine/topiramate in obese and overweight adults (SEQUEL): a randomized, placebo-con-trolled, phase 3 extension study. Am J Clin Nutr. 2012;95:297–308. https://doi.org/10.3945/ajcn.111.024927.
122. O'Neil PM, Smith SR, Weissman NJ, Fidler MC, Sanchez M, Zhang J, et al. Randomized placebo-controlled clinical trial of lorcaserin for weight loss in type 2 diabetes mellitus: the BLOOM-DM study. Obesity (Silver Spring). 2012;20(7):1426–36.
123. Apovian CM, Aronne L, Rubino D, Still C, Wyatt H, Burns C, et al. A randomized, phase 3 trial of naltrexone SR/bupropion SR on weight and obesity-related risk factors (COR-II). Obesity (Silver Spring). 2013;21(5):935–43.
124. Hollander P, Gupta AK, Plodkowski R, Greenway F, Bays H, Burns C, et al. Effects of naltrexone sustained-release/bupropion sustained-release combination therapy on body weight and glycemic parameters in overweight and obese patients with type 2 diabetes. Diabetes Care. 2013;36(12):4022–9.
125. Pi-Sunyer X, Astrup A, Fujioka K, Greenway F, Halpern A, Krempf M, et al. A randomized, controlled trial of 3.0 mg of liraglutide in weight management. N Engl J Med. 2015;373:11–22.
126. Davies MJ, et al. Efficacy of liraglutide for weight loss among patients with type 2 diabetes: the SCALE Diabetes randomized clinical trial. JAMA. 2015;314:687–99.
127. Wadden TA, Hollander P, Klein S, Niswender K, Woo V, Hale PM, et al. Weight maintenance and additional weight loss with liraglutide after low-calorie-diet-induced weight loss: the SCALE Maintenance randomized study. Int J Obes. 2013;37(11):1443–51.
128. le Roux CW, Astrup A, Fujioka K, Greenway F, Lau DCW, Van Gaal L, Ortiz RV, Wilding JPH, Skjøth TV, Manning LS, Pi-Sunyer X, SCALE Obesity Prediabetes NN8022–1839 Study Group. 3 years of liraglutide versus placebo for type 2 diabetes risk reduction and weight management in individuals with prediabetes: a randomised, double-blind trial. Lancet. 2017;389:1399–409. https://doi.org/10.1016/S0140-6736(17)30069-7.
129. Maslov DL, Balashova EE, Lokhov PG, Archakov AI. Pharmacometabonomics—the novel way to personalized drug therapy [Russian]. Biomed Khim. 2017;63:115–23.
130. Adkins DE, et al. Genotype-based ancestral background consistently predicts efficacy and side effects across treatments in CATIE and STAR*D. PLoS One. 2013;8:e55239.
131. Rothman RB, Baumann MH, Savage JE, Rauser L, McBride A, Hufeisen SJ, et al. Evidence for possible involvement of 5-HT(2B) in the cardiac valvulopathy associated with fenfluramine and other serotonergic medications. Circulation. 2000;102(23):2836–41.
132. Rucker D, Padwal R, Li SK, Curioni C, Lau DCW. Long term pharmacotherapy for obesity and overweight: updated meta-analysis. BMJ. 2007;335(7631):1194–9.
133. Johansson K, Sundstrom J, Neovius K, Rossner S, Neovius M. Long-term changes in blood pressure following orlistat and sibutramine treatment: a meta-analysis. Obes Rev. 2010;11(11):777–91.
134. Colman E. Anorectics on trial: a half century of federal regulation of prescription appetite suppressants. Ann Intern Med. 2005;143(5):380–5.
135. Glazer G. Long-term pharmacotherapy of obesity 2000: a review of efficacy and safety. Arch Intern Med. 2001;161:1814–24.
136. Ioannides-Demos LL, Piccenna L, McNeil JJ. Pharmacotherapies for obesity: past, current, and future therapies. J Obes. 2011;2011:179674.
137. Kang JG, Park CY, Kang JH, Park YW, Park SW. Randomized controlled trial to investigate the effects of a newly developed formulation of phentermine diffuse-controlled release for obesity. Diabetes Obes Metab. 2010;12:876–82.
138. Kim KK, Cho HJ, Kang HC, Youn BB, Lee KR. Effects on weight reduction and safety of short-term phentermine administration in korean obese people. Yonsei Med J. 2006;47:614–25.
139. Frank A. The long-term management of obesity with continuing pharmacotherapy. Obes Res. 2004;12:1821–7.

140. Hendricks EJ, Greenway FL, Westman EC, Gupta AK. Blood pressure and heart rate effects, weight loss and maintenance during long-term phentermine pharmacotherapy for obesity. Obesity (Silver Spring). 2011;19:2351–60.
141. Rothman RB. Treatment of obesity with 'combination' pharmacotherapy. Am J Ther. 2010;17:596–603.
142. Hendricks EJ, Rothman RB, Greenway FL. How physician obesity specialists use drugs to treat obesity. Obesity (Silver Spring). 2009;17:1730–5.
143. Hendricks EJ, Greenway FL. A study of abrupt phentermine cessation in patients in a weight management program. Am J Ther. 2011;18:292–9.
144. Gossop M, Darke S, Griffiths P, Hando J, Powis B, Hall W, et al. The Severity of Dependence Scale (SDS): psychometric properties of the SDS in English and Australian samples of heroin, cocaine and amphetamine users. Addiction. 1995;90:607–14.
145. Kelly AS, Fox CK, Rudser KD, Gross AC, Ryder JR. Pediatric obesity pharmacotherapy: current state of the field, review of the literature, and clinical trial considerations. Int J Obes. 2016;40:1043–50.
146. Barlow SE. Expert committee recommendations regarding the prevention, assessment, and treatment of child and adolescent overweight and obesity: summary report. Pediatrics. 2007;120:S164–92.
147. Stafford RS, Radley DC. National trends in antiobesity medication use. Arch Intern Med. 2003;163:1046–50.
148. Calle EE, Thun MJ, Petrelli JM, Rodriguez C, Heath W Jr. Body-mass index and mortality in a prospective cohort of US adults. N Engl J Med. 1999;341:1097–105.
149. Winter Y, Rohrmann S, Linseisen J, Lanczik O, Ringleb PA, Hebebrand J, et al. Contribution of obesity and abdominal fat mass to risk of stroke and transient ischemic attacks. Stroke. 2008;39:3145–51.
150. Cercato C, Mancini MC, Arguello AM, Passos VQ, Villares SM, Halpern A. Systemic hypertension, diabetes mellitus, and dyslipidemia in relation to body mass index: evaluation of a Brazilian population. Rev Hosp Clin Fac Med Sao Paulo. 2004;59:113–8.
151. Haddock CK, Poston WS, Dill PL, Foreyt JP, Ericsson M. Pharmacotherapy for obesity: a quantitative analysis of four decades of published randomized clinical trials. Int J Obes Relat Metab Disord. 2002;26:262–73.
152. Padwal R, Li S, Lau D. Long-term pharmacotherapy for overweight and obesity: a systematic review and meta-analysis of randomized controlled trials. Int J Obes Relat Metab Disord. 2003;27:1437–46.
153. Koliaki C, Dalamaga M, Liatis S. Update on the obesity epidemic: after the sudden rise, is the upward trajectory beginning to flatten? Curr Obes Rep. 2023; https://doi.org/10.1007/s13679-023-00527-y.
154. Pearson-Stuttard J, Banerji T, Capucci S, de Laguiche E, Faurby MD, Haase CL, Sommer Matthiessen K, Near AM, Tse J, Zhao X, Evans M. Real-world costs of obesity-related complications over eight years: a US retrospective cohort study in 28,500 individuals. Int J Obes. 2023; https://doi.org/10.1038/s41366-023-01376-4.
155. Busetto L, Carbonelli MG, Caretto A, Colao A, Cricelli C, De Luca M, Giorgino F, Gnessi L, Medea G, Pappagallo G, Santini F, Sbraccia P, Zappa MA. Updating obesity management strategies: an audit of Italian specialists. Eat Weight Disord. 2022; https://doi.org/10.1007/s40519-022-01402-w.
156. Müller TD, Blüher M, Tschöp MH, DiMarchi RD. Anti-obesity drug discovery: advances and challenges. Nat Rev Drug Discov. 2021; https://doi.org/10.1038/s41573-021-00337-8.
157. Bocarsly ME. Pharmacological interventions for obesity: current and future targets. Curr Addict Rep. 2018; https://doi.org/10.1007/s40429-018-0204-0.
158. Jones BJ, Bloom SR. The new era of drug therapy for obesity: the evidence and the expectations. Drugs. 2015; https://doi.org/10.1007/s40265-015-0410-1.
159. Srivastava G, Apovian CM. Current pharmacotherapy for obesity. Nat Rev Endocrinol. 2017; https://doi.org/10.1038/nrendo.2017.122.

160. Tak YJ, Lee SY. Long-term efficacy and safety of anti-obesity treatment: where do we stand? Curr Obes Rep. 2021; https://doi.org/10.1007/s13679-020-00422-w.
161. Wittert G. Sibutramine and Rimonabant: a Postmortem forensic examination. In: Controversies in obesity; 2013. https://doi.org/10.1007/978-1-4471-2834-2_28.
162. Hendricks EJ, Srisurapanont M, Schmidt SL, Haggard M, Souter S, Mitchell CL, De Marco DG, Hendricks MJ, Istratiy Y, Greenway FL. Addiction potential of phentermine prescribed during long-term treatment of obesity. Int J Obes. 2013; https://doi.org/10.1038/ijo.2013.74.
163. Ryder JR, Kaizer A, Rudser KD, Gross A, Kelly AS, Fox CK. Effect of phentermine on weight reduction in a pediatric weight management clinic. Int J Obes. 2016; https://doi.org/10.1038/ijo.2016.185.
164. Cercato C, Roizenblatt VA, Leança CC, Segal A, Lopes Filho AP, Mancini MC, Halpern A. A randomized double-blind placebo-controlled study of the long-term efficacy and safety of diethylpropion in the treatment of obese subjects. Int J Obes. 2009; https://doi.org/10.1038/ijo.2009.124.

Chapter 2
Orlistat: A Gastrointestinal Lipase Inhibitor

Shilpa Chugh Garcha and Sanjay Kalra

Orlistat is a USFDA-approved weight loss drug that can be used for long-term. Orlistat is a gastrointestinal lipase inhibitor that selectively inhibits the gastric & pancreatic lipases, which leads to decreased fat absorption and increased fecal fat excretion. This mechanism of action helps in weight loss and reducing visceral fat [1].

Many clinical trials and reviews are available that explore the efficacy and safety of orlistat and its effects on various body parameters along with its effect on body fat and weight loss.

This chapter includes studies that explores the efficacy and the safety of orlistat in patients with obesity and the maintenance of weight loss when used over the long term. Some studies also include the effects of orlistat on plasma lipid levels, glycemic indices, blood pressure, and plasma levels of fat-soluble vitamins such as vitamin D.

Studies also observed the effects of orlistat on visceral fat, waist circumference, and further reduction of metabolic disease risk factors.

The efficacy of orlistat has also been explored in patients with hypercholesterolemia and coronary artery disease where orlistat demonstrated weight loss and lowering of LDL cholesterol levels, highlighting its potential in lowering cardiovascular health risk. However, a rebound effect has also been noticed once orlistat is stopped and hence continued treatment may be needed for long-term benefits.

A retrospective analysis pooled data from two large European multicenter trials over two years also assesses the long-term outcomes of orlistat treatment and suggested that an early response to orlistat is an indicator of sustained weight loss and may help in improving obesity-related health conditions.

S. C. Garcha (✉)
Sonepat, Haryana, India

S. Kalra
Department of Endocrinology, Bharti Hospital, Karnal, Haryana, India

S. C. Garcha, S. Kalra (eds.), *Drugs for Medical Management of Obesity*,
https://doi.org/10.1007/978-981-96-1651-0_2

Studies are also investigating the effect of over-the-counter use of 60 mg orlistat on intra-abdominal adipose tissue and ectopic fat highlighting the potential of orlistat 60 mg as an accessible intervention in some communities.

The use of orlistat has been studied in the adolescent population suggesting pharmacological intervention possibilities in childhood obesity along with keeping in view the side effects. Studies also emphasized the need for monitoring of vitamin D levels. A recent meta-analysis of the effects of orlistat on anthropometric and metabolic indices in children and adolescents suggests that even though orlistat reduced the waist circumference and insulin levels in overweight and obese individuals, statistically significant effects were not seen on weight loss, BMI reduction, blood glucose levels, and lipid profile, which contrasts with the results seen in the adult population. This study suggests large sample long term future studies to establish the role of orlistat in weight management for pediatric population.

Benefit-risk assessment of the use of orlistat done by conducting an extensive literature search through databases in one study has highlighted the clinical effectiveness of orlistat and the common gastrointestinal adverse effects of orlistat which may affect compliance. The safety profile of orlistat has also been discussed in a prescription event monitoring study wherein the gastrointestinal side effects were similar as seen in clinical trials. Other safety concerns that were raised included hypersensitivity reactions, and cardiovascular and hepatobiliary events, however, their association was uncertain due to other confounding factors.

We also included one study that investigated the use of natural fibers (psyllium mucilloid) for the prevention of gastrointestinal adverse events when used concomitantly with orlistat.

A case report of pancreatitis with normal amylase levels is included. It hypothesizes orlistat as a cause of pancreatitis while excluding other possible causes of pancreatitis. The authors suggested that many cases of pancreatitis may not be diagnosed due to normal amylase levels, hence pancreatitis should be considered in patients taking orlistat and presenting with abdominal pain. As per the FDA label of orlistat, there have been postmarketing reports of pancreatitis with orlistat, however, no causal relationship has been established between the two (1).

Effects of orlistat on bone health have been explored in a study wherein authors monitored the bone mineral content (BMC) and bone mineral density (BMD) and found that orlistat does not significantly compromise BMC or BMD, even though there was some increase in markers of bone resorption. Vitamin D and calcium supplementation was advised along with orlistat treatment.

A cost-effectiveness study of orlistat utilized a decision model to simulate the health outcomes and costs associated with orlistat plus diet versus diet alone with data from five clinical trials. The study suggested that the average incremental cost per quality-adjusted life year (QALY) gained was within acceptable limits.

More studies on the cost-effectiveness of the use of orlistat would be welcome as obesity and obesity related complications have high economic implications and it is important to see how the use of orlistat can help to manage obesity, prevent the related complications, and hence lower the associated economic burden.

There are many studies available that explore the efficacy and safety of orlistat. More studies to explore the effects of orlistat on various body parameters in pediatric population are needed that can help to establish the role of orlistat as a safe and effective option in the management of obesity in the young population.

Orlistat is generally considered for long-term management of obesity; hence, more studies are needed that can explore its full potential as a safe and effective agent in the management of obesity and its role in preventing obesity-related complications over long-term.

References for Introduction

[1] Xenical (Orlistat). U.S. Food and Drug Administration website. https://www.accessdata.fda.gov/drugsatfda_docs/label/2022/020766s038lbl.pdf. Revised August 2016. Accessed 6 Aug 2024

2.1 Machine Generated Summaries

Disclaimer: The summaries in this chapter were generated from Springer Nature publications using abstractive AI auto-summarization: An abstraction-based summarizer creates new text based on deep learning. New phrases are created to summarize the content. As the constituted sentences are machine selected, they may not fully reflect the body of the work, so we strongly advise that the original content is read and cited. The auto-generated summaries were curated by the editor to meet Springer Nature publication standards.

Machine generated keywords: orlistat, orlistat treatment, obese patient, dietary fat, body composition, cholesterol.

Spotlight on Orlistat in the Management of Patients with Obesity [118]

This is a machine-generated summary of:

Curran, Monique P.; Scott, Lesley J.: Spotlight on Orlistat in the Management of Patients with Obesity [118]

Published in: Treatments in Endocrinology (2005)

Link to original: https://doi.org/10.2165/00024677-200504020-00006

If you want to cite the papers, please refer to the original.

For technical reasons we could not place the page where the original quote is coming from.

Research highlights

Obesity is a global health concern associated with numerous comorbidities, including type 2 diabetes, hypertension, and cardiovascular disease. Despite the availability of various weight management strategies, there remains a significant gap in effective long-term pharmacological interventions. Now a new study by

Monique P. Curran and Lesley J Scott sheds light on the efficacy and safety of orlistat, a drug that inhibits fat absorption, as a promising therapeutic option for obesity management.

The authors evaluated orlistat's pharmacologic properties and therapeutic use in obese patients. By selectively inhibiting gastric and pancreatic lipases, orlistat prevents the hydrolysis and subsequent absorption of dietary fats, leading to increased fecal fat excretion without affecting fat-free mass or resting energy expenditure. The study highlighted orlistat's role in improving metabolic parameters such as plasma lipid levels, measurement of glycemic control, plasma leptin, hemostatic factors, and blood pressure. The XENDOS trial, a cornerstone of their analysis, demonstrated that orlistat not only significantly reduced body weight over four years but also decreased the risk of developing type 2 diabetes mellitus by 37.3% as compared to placebo. The researchers employed rigorous methodologies, including large-scale trials and long-term cost-effectiveness analyses, to substantiate their findings. The study suggests that orlistat's minimal absorption and rapid elimination profile underscore its suitability for long-term administration.

The main advances from this study include orlistat's significant impact on weight reduction and metabolic risk factors in obese patients with comorbidities such as type 2 diabetes. Moreover, the drug was found to be cost-effective for managing obesity-related conditions. While gastrointestinal side effects were the most commonly reported adverse events, they were typically mild and transient. Curran suggests that "The tolerability and sustained efficacy of orlistat make it an invaluable component in the obesity treatment arsenal."

Weight Reduction and Long-Term Maintenance After 18 Months Treatment with Orlistat for Obesity [119]

This is a machine-generated summary of:

Krempf, M; Louvet, J-P; Allanic, H; Miloradovich, T; Joubert, J-M; Attali, J-R: Weight reduction and long-term maintenance after 18 months treatment with orlistat for obesity [119]

Published in: International Journal of Obesity (2003)

Link to original: https://doi.org/10.1038/sj.ijo.0802281

If you want to cite the papers, please refer to the original.

For technical reasons we could not place the page where the original quote is coming from.

Research highlights

Introduction:

The global rise in obesity has been linked to increased risks of coronary heart disease, type II diabetes, dyslipidemia, and hypertension. Despite the urgent need for effective weight management strategies, traditional dietary and behavioral interventions often fail to produce sustained weight loss. Now a new study by M Krempf and colleagues addresses this challenge by examining the long-term efficacy of orlistat, a lipase inhibitor that reduces dietary fat absorption, in combination with a continuous mildly reduced-energy diet over an 18-month period.

In this groundbreaking research, men and women with a body mass index (BMI) of 28 kg/m^2 or higher were recruited, excluding those with serious eating disorders or other significant health issues. The study adhered to ethical guidelines and participants provided informed consent. A double-blind, randomized, placebo-controlled trial design was employed across several French hospital centers. Participants were assigned to receive either orlistat or a placebo alongside tailored dietary advice aimed at reducing energy intake by 20% and limiting fat intake to 30% of energy intake. Food diaries were used to monitor compliance and adjust dietary plans accordingly. Weight, BMI, body fat, and various health markers were measured at regular intervals to assess the impact of the treatment.

The results revealed that patients on orlistat experienced significantly greater weight loss compared to those on the placebo. Notably, the orlistat group maintained this weight loss more effectively over the 18-month period. The study also found that early responders to orlistat treatment showed particularly impressive weight loss results. Furthermore, while both groups saw reductions in body fat mass, the decrease was more pronounced in those taking orlistat.

Conclusion:

M Krempf's study marks a significant advance in obesity treatment by demonstrating that long-term weight loss can be achieved with orlistat in conjunction with a consistent reduced-energy diet. The findings suggest that this combination not only facilitates initial weight loss but also aids in maintaining it over an extended period.

Reduction of Excessive Visceral Fat and Safety with 52-Week Administration of Lipase Inhibitor Orlistat in Japanese: Long-Term Clinical Study [120]

This is a machine-generated summary of:

Shirai, Kohji; Tanaka, Michitaka; Fujita, Toru; Fujii, Yuka; Shimomasuda, Masatsugu; Sakai, Soichi; Samukawa, Yoshishige: Reduction of Excessive Visceral Fat and Safety with 52-Week Administration of Lipase Inhibitor Orlistat in Japanese: Long-Term Clinical Study [120].

Published in: Advances in Therapy (2018)

Link to original: https://doi.org/10.1007/s12325-018-0822-x

If you want to cite the papers, please refer to the original.

For technical reasons we could not place the page where the original quote is coming from.

Research highlights

Introduction:

The global rise in obesity has been linked to an array of health complications, including metabolic disorders and cardiovascular diseases. Despite lower overall obesity rates, Japan faces a high incidence of obesity-related conditions, suggesting that even mild obesity can lead to significant health issues. A key factor in this is the accumulation of visceral fat, which is more closely associated with metabolic diseases than subcutaneous fat. Now a new study by Kohji Shirai and colleagues addresses the efficacy and safety of long-term orlistat administration in Japanese individuals with excessive visceral fat but without metabolic diseases, offering insights into potential treatments for obesity-related health risks.

Body:

Shirai et al.'s research involved an open-label, uncontrolled study over 52 weeks with Japanese participants who had excessive visceral fat accumulation but no metabolic diseases. The participants were administered 60 mg of orlistat three times daily alongside dietary improvements and consistent exercise habits. The study's design included regular interviews, body measurements, blood pressure assessments, and clinical laboratory testing to monitor the effects of the treatment.

The results were promising: significant reductions in visceral fat area, waist circumference, and body weight were observed throughout the treatment period. Moreover, the study reported improvements in lipid profiles and a decrease in the number of metabolic disease risk factors among participants. The authors noted that while orlistat's primary action is to inhibit dietary fat absorption, it may also enhance lipid utilization within the body, contributing to these positive outcomes.

Conclusion:

The main advances highlighted by Shirai et al.'s study include the confirmation that long-term administration of orlistat can significantly reduce visceral fat and waist circumference in a Japanese population without causing severe side effects. This suggests that orlistat could be a valuable tool for managing obesity-related health risks through its ability to complement lifestyle changes such as diet and exercise. Looking forward, these findings pave the way for considering orlistat as an early intervention strategy in obesity management. As Shirai et al. conclude, "The longer orlistat is administered, the more visceral fat is expected to decrease; moreover, it may lead to reductions in risk factors for metabolic diseases caused by obesity," indicating a promising future direction for obesity treatment strategies.

The Effects of Orlistat on Weight and on Serum Lipids in Obese Patients with Hypercholesterolemia: A Randomized, Double-Blind, Placebo-Controlled, Multicentre Study [121]

This is a machine-generated summary of:

Muls, E; Kolanowski, J; Scheen, A; Van Gaal, L: The effects of orlistat on weight and on serum lipids in obese patients with hypercholesterolemia: a randomized, double-blind, placebo-controlled, multicentre study [121].

Published in: International Journal of Obesity (2001)

Link to original: https://doi.org/10.1038/sj.ijo.0801814

If you want to cite the papers, please refer to the original.

For technical reasons we could not place the page where the original quote is coming from.

Research highlights

Research Highlight

Dyslipidemia, characterized by abnormal lipid levels in the blood, is closely linked to obesity and significantly increases the risk of coronary heart disease. While lifestyle changes such as diet and exercise can mitigate these risks, maintaining weight loss is notoriously challenging, necessitating additional pharmacological interventions. Now a new study by E. Muls and colleagues has explored the efficacy of orlistat, a lipase inhibitor that reduces dietary fat absorption, in promoting weight loss and improving serum lipid profiles in obese patients with hypercholesterolemia.

In this 50 week, multicenter, randomized, placebo-controlled trial, obese patients with elevated LDL cholesterol levels were assigned to receive either orlistat or a placebo alongside a hypocaloric diet. The study's design included an initial run-in phase followed by a double-blind phase and an open-label extension with orlistat. Patients' adherence to the treatment regimen was monitored through clinic visits and dietary compliance assessments. The primary outcomes measured were changes in body weight and serum lipid levels, analyzed using various statistical methods to ensure robustness of the findings.

The results demonstrated that orlistat significantly enhanced weight loss compared to placebo and led to additional reductions in LDL cholesterol levels independent of weight loss. These findings suggest that orlistat not only aids in achieving weight loss but also contributes to lowering cardiovascular risk factors in obese individuals with hypercholesterolemia. Looking forward, these results underscore the potential for orlistat as an adjunct therapy along with dietary intervention for long-term weight management and LDL-C reduction. As E. Muls et al. conclude, the drug's favorable impact on lipid profiles extends its benefits beyond mere weight control.

The Effects of Diet and Orlistat on Body Weight and Lipid Profiles in High Risk Chinese Patients with Coronary Artery Disease, Obesity and Hypercholesterolemia [122]

This is a machine-generated summary of:

Chan, K. W.; Leung, W. S.; Fung, Y. S.; Hung, H. F.; Tsui, P.; Chu, H.; Chan, Y. W.; Ko, G. T. C.; Yeung, V. T. F.: The effects of diet and orlistat on body weight and lipid profiles in high risk Chinese patients with coronary artery disease, obesity and hypercholesterolemia [122]

Published in: Irish Journal of Medical Science (2009)

Link to original: https://doi.org/10.1007/s11845-009-0291-y

If you want to cite the papers, please refer to the original.

For technical reasons we could not place the page where the original quote is coming from.

Research highlights

Introduction:

Coronary artery disease (CAD) remains a leading cause of mortality worldwide, with lifestyle changes contributing to its prevalence. In Hong Kong, the mortality rate from CAD has seen a dramatic increase, correlating with rising obesity and hypercholesterolemia rates. Despite lifestyle recommendations, adherence to dietary restrictions is waning, underscoring the need for additional interventions. Now a new study by K.W. Chan and colleagues addresses this challenge by examining the impact of orlistat, a gastrointestinal lipase inhibitor, on weight and lipid management in non-diabetic Chinese patients with established CAD.

Main Body:

The study enrolled thirty Chinese patients from the Medical and Geriatric Clinics of a general hospital in Hong Kong who met specific inclusion criteria, such as confirmed CAD and a body mass index (BMI) ≥ 25 kg/m^2. The research design included a 12-week dietary control phase followed by 24 weeks of orlistat treatment at 120 mg thrice daily with meals. Chan et al. meticulously monitored body weight, lipid profiles, blood pressure, fasting blood glucose levels, and adverse reactions throughout the study period.

Statistical analysis revealed significant reductions in body weight and improvements in lipid profiles during the orlistat phase. However, upon cessation of orlistat for 12 weeks, some benefits were reversed, indicating the importance of continued treatment for sustained effects. The authors emphasized that the overall effect of 12-week dietary treatment followed by 24-week dietary and orlistat treatment resulted in significant reduction of body weight by 4.6% and BMI by 4.5%, showcasing the potential of orlistat as an adjunct therapy for weight and lipid management in CAD patients.

Conclusion:

The study by Chan et al. marks a significant advance in understanding how pharmacotherapy can complement lifestyle changes in managing CAD risk factors. The findings suggest that orlistat effectively promotes weight loss and improves lipid profiles in obese non-diabetic Chinese patients with established CAD. While there was a rebound effect after stopping orlistat, the research supports its use as part of a comprehensive treatment plan for CAD patients struggling with obesity and hypercholesterolemia.

Chan reflects on the broader implications and suggests that this independent cholesterol-lowering effect is likely to be beneficial to our patients with established CAD. Looking forward, controlled studies could further validate these results. The study paves the way for integrating pharmacological agents like orlistat into standard care for CAD patients to enhance secondary prevention efforts.

Predictive Value of Early Weight Loss in Obesity Management with Orlistat: an Evidence-Based Assessment of Prescribing Guidelines [123]

This is a machine-generated summary of:

Rissanen, A; Lean, M; Rössner, S; Segal, K R; Sjöström, L: Predictive value of early weight loss in obesity management with orlistat: an evidence-based assessment of prescribing guidelines [123]

Published in: International Journal of Obesity (2003)
Link to original: https://doi.org/10.1038/sj.ijo.0802165

If you want to cite the papers, please refer to the original.

For technical reasons we could not place the page where the original quote is coming from.

Research highlights

Introduction:

Obesity is a global health concern, with weight loss of 5–10% known to improve related cardiovascular and metabolic abnormalities. However, maintaining weight loss through conventional methods often fails, prompting interest in pharmacotherapy as an adjunct. Identifying patients who will benefit from such treatments is crucial for enhancing outcomes and minimizing risks. Clinical trials suggest that early responders to pharmacotherapy are likely to continue benefiting, while non-responders remain so. Yet, evidence-based guidelines for pharmacotherapy in obesity are lacking.

Now a new study by A Rissanen and colleagues addresses this gap by examining the effectiveness of orlistat, a gastrointestinal lipase inhibitor and evaluating the validity of current prescribing recommendations.

Main Body:

Rissanen et al.'s retrospective analysis pooled data from two large two-year European multicenter trials to assess the long-term outcomes of orlistat treatment. The study involved overweight and obese adults who underwent a lead-in period with a hypocaloric diet before being randomized to receive either orlistat or placebo alongside continued dietary intervention. The researchers focused on patients who completed the full two-year treatment with orlistat, analyzing weight loss and secondary efficacy parameters such as serum lipid concentrations, blood pressure, fasting serum glucose and insulin concentrations.

The study's design allowed for an evaluation of whether early weight loss during orlistat treatment could predict sustained benefits. The authors found that patients who lost ≥5% of their body weight after 12 weeks of drug therapy were more likely to maintain significant weight loss after two years, supporting the criteria set by European prescribing information and recent guidance from the National Institute for Clinical Excellence (NICE).

Conclusion:

The findings by Rissanen et al. represent a significant advance in understanding the long-term benefits of pharmacotherapy for obesity management. The study confirms that an early response to orlistat is predictive of sustained weight loss and improvement in obesity-related health conditions. Looking forward, these insights may inform future clinical practice guidelines, ensuring that patients most likely to benefit from pharmacotherapy receive appropriate treatment while minimizing unnecessary exposure for non-responders.

Pragmatic Study of Orlistat 60 mg on Abdominal Obesity [124]

This is a machine-generated summary of:

Thomas, E L; Makwana, A; Newbould, R; Rao, A W; Gambarota, G; Frost, G; Delafont, B; Mishra, R G; Matthews, P M; Berk, E S; Schwartz, S M; Bell, J D; Beaver, J D: Pragmatic study of orlistat 60 mg on abdominal obesity [124]

Published in: European Journal of Clinical Nutrition (2011)

Link to original: https://doi.org/10.1038/ejcn.2011.108

If you want to cite the papers, please refer to the original.

For technical reasons we could not place the page where the original quote is coming from.

Research highlights

Introduction:

The global obesity epidemic poses a significant challenge to healthcare systems, with limited long-term pharmacological interventions available. Despite the demonstrated efficacy of orlistat 60 mg in reducing body weight and of orlistat 120 mg in improving body composition, the impact of orlistat 60 mg on weight loss and body composition in a real-world community setting remains unclear. Now a new study by E L Thomas and colleagues addresses this gap by investigating the effects of over-the-counter orlistat 60 mg given for 12 weeks on body composition, specifically targeting intra-abdominal adipose tissue (IAAT) and ectopic fat, in overweight and obese individuals within a free-living community.

Main Body:

Thomas et al. conducted an open-label, non-randomized 12-week study without a control group to mimic the conditions of actual over-the-counter medication use. The study recruited 27 subjects through local advertising and recruited individuals from local prisons and police forces, resulting in a male-biased sample. Participants were provided with orlistat 60 mg and educational materials similar to those included in the US starter kit for alli®, along with access to the US alli website. The researchers employed both MRI and H MR spectroscopy imaging to measure changes in IAAT and ectopic fat after the treatment period. The methods were thorough: subjects underwent physical exams, routine safety tests, and dietary assessments using a multipass 24-hour recall analyzed with Dietplan6 software. MRI scans assessed abdominal subcutaneous adipose tissue (ASAT) and IAAT, while MRS measured liver and soleus muscle lipid content.

Statistical analyses accounted for baseline characteristics, age, gender, and used analyses of covariance to present relative changes from baseline.

Conclusion:

The study by Thomas et al. reveals that even with minimal professional guidance typical of an over-the-counter setting, orlistat 60 mg can lead to significant reductions in IAAT and ectopic fat after 12 weeks. The intervention also resulted in notable decreases in body weight, waist circumference (WC), BMI, and improvements in blood lipid profiles, liver function tests, and blood pressure—markers associated with reduced risk factors for metabolic diseases.

These findings underscore the potential of orlistat 60 mg as an accessible intervention for weight management in community settings. The authors also observed reductions in pericardial fat volumes and intrahepatic lipids. While the study did not include a control group due to its real-world design, the results align with previous research on orlistat's efficacy.

Addition of Orlistat to Conventional Treatment in Adolescents with Severe Obesity [125]

This is a machine-generated summary of:

Ozkan, Behzat; Bereket, Abdullah; Turan, Serap; Keskin, Sabiha: Addition of orlistat to conventional treatment in adolescents with severe obesity [125]

Published in: European Journal of Pediatrics (2004)

Link to original: https://doi.org/10.1007/s00431-004-1534-6

If you want to cite the papers, please refer to the original.

For technical reasons we could not place the page where the original quote is coming from.

Research highlights

Research Highlight

Childhood obesity is a growing concern worldwide, leading to an increase in related health issues such as type 2 diabetes, sleep apnoea, hypertension, orthopaedic problems, and others.

Despite efforts to manage obesity through behavioral therapy by dietary and physical activity modifications, the success rates remain low due to challenges in maintaining hypocaloric diet in children. Now a new study by Behzat Ozkan and colleagues addresses this issue by exploring the efficacy and tolerability of orlistat, a gastrointestinal lipase inhibitor, in obese adolescents.

Ozkan's team conducted a prospective, open-controlled pilot study with subjects aged 10–16 years who were severely obese but otherwise healthy. The study compared conventional treatment alone to conventional treatment combined with orlistat.

Participants were monitored for weight, and body mass index (BMI). Patients in the orlistat group also received a daily multivitamin. Despite similar compliance rates for diet and exercise between groups, the orlistat group showed significant weight loss and BMI reduction compared to the control group, which saw weight gain on average. However, gastrointestinal complaints led to a dropout rate of about one-third in the orlistat group.

The study highlights that while orlistat can be an effective adjunct to lifestyle interventions for weight loss in adolescents, its use is limited by tolerability issues. The authors suggest that future research should focus on larger placebo-controlled studies to better understand the long-term benefits and risks of orlistat in pediatric populations. They also emphasize the need for close monitoring of vitamin D levels due to potential reductions caused by orlistat treatment. This research opens up new possibilities for pharmacological intervention in childhood obesity but also underscores the importance of addressing associated side effects.

Effect of Orlistat on Anthropometrics and Metabolic Indices in Children and Adolescents: A Systematic Review and Meta-Analysis [126]

This is a machine-generated summary of:

Nikniaz, Zeinab; Nikniaz, Leila; Farhangi, Mahdieh Abbasalizad; Mehralizadeh, Hossein; Salekzamani, Shabnam: Effect of Orlistat on anthropometrics and metabolic indices in children and adolescents: a systematic review and meta-analysis [126]

Published in: BMC Endocrine Disorders (2023)

Link to original: https://doi.org/10.1186/s12902-023-01390-7

If you want to cite the papers, please refer to the original.

For technical reasons we could not place the page where the original quote is coming from.

Research highlights

Childhood obesity has emerged as a global epidemic, with millions of children over five years old being overweight or obese in 2016, a figure that has quadrupled since the 1975s. This alarming trend is not only associated with immediate health complications in children but also predisposes them to chronic diseases in adulthood. Despite the known benefits of diet and exercise, their effectiveness in managing pediatric obesity has been underwhelming. Now a new study by Zeinab Nikniaz and colleagues addresses this critical issue by systematically reviewing the impact of Orlistat, an FDA-approved anti-obesity medication for adolescents, on weight loss and other metabolic parameters in this demographic.

Nikniaz et al.'s research utilized the Preferred Reporting Items for Systematic Review and Meta-analysis (PRISMA) guidelines to ensure rigorous methodology. The team conducted a comprehensive search across PubMed, Scopus, and Web of Science databases, meticulously screening for studies that met their inclusion criteria. They focused on experimental and semi-experimental studies that reported on Orlistat's effects on obesity-related parameters in children. The meta-analysis incorporated data from four experimental studies and two semi-experimental studies, assessing outcomes such as weight, BMI, lipid profiles, fasting blood glucose, and insulin levels. The authors carefully evaluated the risk of bias within these studies using a revised Cochrane risk-of-bias tool and resolved any discrepancies through consensus.

The study's findings are nuanced; while Orlistat significantly reduced waist circumference and insulin levels in overweight and obese adolescents, its effects on weight loss, BMI reduction, blood glucose levels, and lipid profile improvements were not statistically significant. These results contrast with those observed in adult populations where Orlistat has demonstrated more pronounced benefits. The authors suggest that future research should consider longer-term studies with larger sample sizes to fully ascertain Orlistat's role in treating pediatric obesity. Additionally, they recommend that future trials take into account potential drug-drug interactions due to Orlistat's mechanism of action.

In summary, Zeinab Nikniaz et al.'s systematic review highlights the potential of Orlistat as a pharmacological intervention for reducing certain metabolic risk factors associated with adolescent obesity. However, its limited impact on overall weight and BMI underscores the need for more comprehensive treatment strategies. This research paves the way for further investigations into effective obesity treatments for young populations at risk of lifelong health consequences.

Benefit-Risk Assessment of Orlistat in the Treatment of Obesity [127]

This is a machine-generated summary of:

Sumithran, Priya; Proietto, Joseph: Benefit-Risk Assessment of Orlistat in the Treatment of Obesity [127]

Published in: Drug Safety (2014)

Link to original: https://doi.org/10.1007/s40264-014-0210-7

If you want to cite the papers, please refer to the original.

For technical reasons we could not place the page where the original quote is coming from.

Research highlights

Introduction:

The global obesity epidemic poses a significant health challenge, with over one-third of adults worldwide being overweight and >10% are obese. Excess weight is a known risk factor for numerous health conditions, including coronary artery disease, hypertension, type 2 diabetes mellitus, osteoarthritis, obstructive sleep apnea, and various cancers. Weight loss of 5–10% can significantly reduce these risks. Orlistat, a gastrointestinal lipase inhibitor available since the late 1990s, aids in obesity management by reducing dietary fat absorption. Now a new study by Priya Sumithran and Joseph Proietto delves into the efficacy and safety of orlistat, providing a comprehensive review of its role in treating obesity. In their research, Sumithran and Proietto conducted an extensive literature search through databases such as MEDLINE and various adverse event reporting systems to gather data on orlistat use between 1987 and 2013. The study meticulously reviewed articles focusing on orlistat's application for obesity treatment, related metabolic conditions or adverse events while excluding off-label uses. The authors synthesized findings from numerous clinical studies and meta-analyses to assess orlistat's impact on body weight regulation, its mode of action, administration guidelines, benefits in weight loss maintenance, effects on blood pressure, lipids, glucose levels, and its use in adolescents.

Sumithran and Proietto highlight that orlistat contributes to modest but clinically significant weight loss and improvements in cardiovascular risk factors including blood pressure, glycemic status, and LDL cholesterol levels. However, they also note the challenges of treatment adherence in real-world settings compared to clinical trials. While serious adverse events like acute kidney or liver injury are rare with orlistat use, gastrointestinal side effects are common and may affect long-term compliance. Looking forward, the authors suggest that despite the availability of newer pharmacotherapies for obesity management in some countries, orlistat remains a valuable option due to its safety profile—particularly for patients with cardiovascular disease or mood disorders. The study underscores the need for individualized treatment plans considering the risks and benefits of available medications.

Safety Profile of Orlistat: Results of a Prescription-Event Monitoring Study [128]

This is a machine-generated summary of:

Acharya, N V; Wilton, L V; Shakir, S A W: Safety profile of orlistat: results of a prescription-event monitoring study [128]

Published in: International Journal of Obesity (2006)

Link to original: https://doi.org/10.1038/sj.ijo.0803323

If you want to cite the papers, please refer to the original.

For technical reasons we could not place the page where the original quote is coming from.

Research highlights

Background and Key Findings:

Orlistat, a lipase inhibitor, has shown promise by preventing the absorption of dietary fats, thereby aiding in weight management when used alongside a reduced-calorie diet. Now a new study by N V Acharya and colleagues provides comprehensive postmarketing surveillance data on orlistat's safety as prescribed by primary care physicians in England.

Study Narrative:

Acharya et al.'s research utilized prescription-event monitoring (PEM), an observational cohort study design, to collect clinical data from patients prescribed orlistat between December 1998 and November 1999. The methodology involved sending questionnaires to GPs, who reported on patient demographics, treatment indication and effectiveness, duration, reasons for discontinuation, and any significant events post-prescription. Events were meticulously coded and assessed for causality using established criteria. The study's robust cohort size enhanced its ability to detect adverse drug reactions (ADRs) with reasonable certainty. Statistical analysis focused on incidence densities of reported events during treatment, revealing that certain events occurred more frequently at the onset (during first month) of orlistat therapy.

Advances and Future Directions:

The study by Acharya et al. marks a significant advance in understanding orlistat's safety profile in primary care settings. It identified specific adverse events associated with the initiation of orlistat treatment, particularly gastrointestinal issues which were consistent with clinical trial observations but occurred at lower rates. Signals for hypersensitivity reactions were also detected and have since been incorporated into the updated prescribing information summary of product characteristics (SPC). The authors note that while some cardiovascular and hepatobiliary concerns were observed, their association with orlistat remains uncertain due to confounding factors related to obesity itself. Looking forward, this research underscores the importance of ongoing post-marketing surveillance to refine our understanding of orlistat's safety and guide its optimal use in managing obesity. As Acharya et al. suggest, "The findings from this study must be placed in context with those of other studies," highlighting the need for continued research to ensure patient safety and drug efficacy.

Gastrointestinal Side Effects of Orlistat May Be Prevented by Concomitant Prescription of Natural Fibers (Psyllium Mucilloid) [129]

This is a machine-generated summary of:

Cavaliere, H; Floriano, I; Medeiros-Neto, G: Gastrointestinal side effects of orlistat may be prevented by concomitant prescription of natural fibers (psyllium mucilloid) [129]

Published in: International Journal of Obesity (2001)

Link to original: https://doi.org/10.1038/sj.ijo.0801645

If you want to cite the papers, please refer to the original.

For technical reasons we could not place the page where the original quote is coming from.

Research highlights

Orlistat, a drug designed to treat obesity, works by inhibiting enzymes that digest fat, leading to reduced fat absorption and increased fat excretion. However, its therapeutic use is often accompanied by gastrointestinal (GI) side effects such as intestinal flatulence, abdominal cramps, fecal incontinence, and oily spotting, which can lead to treatment discontinuation. Now a new study by H Cavaliere and colleagues addresses this issue by investigating the effects of psyllium hydrophilic mucilloid—a soluble fiber known for its beneficial GI properties—on mitigating the adverse effects associated with orlistat therapy.

In their research, Cavaliere et al. conducted a randomized controlled trial involving obese female patients from a university hospital. These participants were divided into two groups: one received orlistat with psyllium, and the other received orlistat with a placebo. The study was meticulously designed to ensure blinding and adherence, with patients reporting their GI events weekly using a scoring system that quantified the severity of symptoms. The researchers found that the group taking psyllium alongside orlistat experienced significantly fewer GI events compared to the placebo group. This effect remained consistent when the groups were switched after a washout period.

The study by Cavaliere's team marks a significant advance in the management of obesity with orlistat. The addition of psyllium not only reduced the frequency and severity of GI side effects but also improved patient convenience and comfort during treatment. As quoted by the authors, "psyllium hydrophilic mucilloid is an effective, practical and easy method to circumvent the GI events during orlistat treatment of obese patients, provided that a moderate fat intake is advised." Looking forward, this research suggests potential for broader applications of dietary fibers in managing medication-induced GI symptoms.

36 Year Old Man Presenting with Pancreatitis and a History of Recent Commencement of Orlistat Case Report [130]

This is a machine-generated summary of:

Napier, Sarah; Thomas, Matthew: 36 year old man presenting with pancreatitis and a history of recent commencement of orlistat case report [130]

Published in: Nutrition Journal (2006)

Link to original: https://doi.org/10.1186/1475-2891-5-19

If you want to cite the papers, please refer to the original.

For technical reasons we could not place the page where the original quote is coming from.

Research highlights

Orlistat, a long-standing anti-obesity drug in the UK, has been associated with various gastrointestinal side effects but not explicitly linked to pancreatitis in clinical trials. Despite its widespread use, the potential for orlistat-induced pancreatitis remains underexplored. Now a new study by Sarah Napier and colleagues presents a compelling case of a patient who developed acute pancreatitis shortly after initiating orlistat treatment, suggesting a possible connection that warrants further investigation.

In this case report, the authors meticulously document the clinical journey of a 36-year-old man with a history of Type II Diabetes Mellitus and other comorbidities including hypertension, asthma, and obstructive sleep apnoea who presented with severe abdominal pain and other symptoms (two episodes of vomiting and loose stool). The patient's recent commencement of orlistat was the only significant change in his medication regimen, leading to the hypothesis that orlistat could be the causative agent. Through careful exclusion of common etiologies such as alcohol consumption and gallstones, and despite normal amylase levels—a marker typically elevated in pancreatitis—the authors diagnosed him with drug-induced pancreatitis secondary to orlistat. The study delves into the diagnostic process, including CT imaging and laboratory tests, and discusses the patient's management in intensive care, which followed standard protocols for treating acute severe pancreatitis.

The main advance highlighted by Napier et al.'s research is the identification of orlistat as a potential cause of pancreatitis even when amylase levels are normal, challenging existing diagnostic paradigms. This finding is particularly significant given that drug-induced pancreatitis is often milder and may go unrecognized if clinicians rely solely on typical biomarkers. The authors call for increased vigilance among healthcare providers when patients present with abdominal pain after starting orlistat, especially in the absence of other risk factors for pancreatitis. As Napier notes, "If orlistat can cause a pancreatitis with normal amylase it is possible that more cases exist but are not fully diagnosed."

Influence of Orlistat on Bone Turnover and Body Composition [131]

This is a machine-generated summary of:

Gotfredsen, A; Westergren Hendel, H; Andersen, T: Influence of orlistat on bone turnover and body composition [131]

Published in: International Journal of Obesity (2001).

Link to original: https://doi.org/10.1038/sj.ijo.0801639

If you want to cite the papers, please refer to the original.

For technical reasons we could not place the page where the original quote is coming from.

Research highlights

Background and Key Findings:

Orlistat (OLS) is a pharmacological agent used to treat obesity by reducing dietary fat absorption, yet its impact on bone health on long term use remains unclear. While obesity is associated with increased bone mass and density, weight loss can lead to a reduction in these parameters, potentially mediated by changes in the function of parathyroid or underlying mechanical load alterations. Now a new study by A Gotfredsen and colleagues investigates the effects of long-term OLS treatment on calcium metabolism and bone mineral content in obese patients, revealing that OLS does not significantly affect bone health over a one-year period.

Study Narrative:

The research conducted by Gotfredsen et al. involved a subset of patients from a larger study, focusing on those who completed one year of treatment. Participants were randomized to receive either OLS or placebo alongside a calorie and fat-restricted diet. Bone mineral content (BMC) and density (BMD) were measured using dual-energy X-ray absorptiometry (DXA), while body composition was assessed through DXA and total body potassium (TBK) counting. Biochemical markers of bone metabolism were also evaluated. The authors found that both groups experienced significant weight loss without significant differences between the groups. Importantly, except the significant changes in forearm measurements, changes in BMC and BMD were minimal and not significantly different between the OLS and placebo groups, suggesting that OLS does not adversely affect these parameters more than that would occur from the weight loss alone.

Advances and Future Directions:

The study's main advance lies in demonstrating that one year of OLS treatment, while promoting weight loss through fat malabsorption, does not significantly compromise bone mineral content or density beyond the effects of weight loss itself. This suggests that OLS can be considered safe for bone health over the studied period. However, Gotfredsen et al. note relative increases in markers of bone resorption in the OLS group, hinting at slightly elevated bone turnover. They recommend vitamin D and calcium supplementation during OLS treatment to mitigate any potential malabsorption issues.

The Cost Effectiveness of Orlistat in a 1-Year Weight-Management Programme for Treating Overweight and Obese Patients in Sweden [132]

This is a machine-generated summary of:

Hertzman, Peter: The cost effectiveness of orlistat in a 1-year weight-management programme for treating overweight and obese patients in Sweden [132]

Published in: PharmacoEconomics (2005)

Link to original: https://doi.org/10.2165/00019053-200523100-00004

Copyright of the summarized publication:

Adis Data Information BV 2005

If you want to cite the papers, please refer to the original.

For technical reasons we could not place the page where the original quote is coming from.

Research highlights

Obesity is a growing health problem throughout the developed world, with a significant rise in prevalence over recent decades. Despite the known risks associated with obesity, including diabetes and cardiovascular diseases, there is a lack of evidence on the cost-effectiveness of weight-loss and weight-maintenance programs. Now a new study by Peter Hertzman addresses this gap by analyzing the cost-effectiveness of orlistat, an oral gastrointestinal lipase inhibitor, as an adjunct to a dietary program compared to diet alone for obese and overweight individuals without diabetes.

Hertzman's research utilized a decision model incorporating data from five pivotal clinical trials to simulate the health outcomes and costs associated with orlistat plus diet versus diet alone. The study focused on patients who were non-diabetic, overweight or obese, and who could achieve at least 2.5 kg weight loss during a lead-in period before receiving orlistat treatment.

The model predicted long-term health states based on initial weight loss and subsequent weight management, considering the impact on type 2 diabetes incidence. The study states that patients treated with orlistat were more likely to achieve significant weight loss compared to those on diet alone and early identification of treatment responders could enhance program cost-effectiveness.

The main advances highlighted by this study include the potential for orlistat to offer a cost-effective solution for managing obesity when used as part of a dietary program. Hertzman estimated an average incremental cost per quality-adjusted life year (QALY) gained that was within acceptable limits for healthcare interventions. The study underscores the importance of using a responder approach in weight management programs to optimize outcomes and resource allocation. Looking forward, the author suggests that future research should focus on long-term effects of weight loss with orlistat and other programs, as well as their impact on cardiovascular risk factors and quality of life.

Bibliography

1. Bakris G, Calhoun D, Egan B, et al. Orlistat improves blood pressure control in obese subjects with treated but inadequately controlled hypertension. J Hypertens. 2002;20(11):2257–67.
2. Broom I, Wilding J, Stott P, et al. Randomised trial of the effect of orlistat on body weight and cardiovascular disease risk profile in obese patients: UK Multi-morbidity Study. Int J Clin Pract. 2002;56(7):494–9.
3. Sjostrom L, Rissanen A, Andersen T, et al. Randomised placebo-controlled trial of orlistat for weight loss and prevention of weight regain in obese patients: European Multicentre Orlistat Study Group. Lancet. 1998;352(9123):167–72.

4. Torgerson JS, Hauptman J, Boldrin MN, Sjöström L. XENical in the prevention of diabetes in obese subjects (XENDOS) study: a randomized study of orlistat as an adjunct to lifestyle changes for the prevention of type 2 diabetes in obese patients. Diabetes Care. 2004;27:155–61.
5. Guy-Grand B, Drouin P, Eschwege E, et al. Effects of orlistat on obesity-related diseases: a six-month randomized trial. Diabetes Obes Metab. 2004;6(5):375–83.
6. Hanefeld M, Sachse G. The effects of orlistat on body weight and glycaemic control in overweight patients with type 2 diabetes: a randomized, placebo-controlled trial. Diabetes Obes Metab. 2002;4(6):415–23.
7. Miles JM, Leiter L, Hollander P, et al. Effect of orlistat in overweight and obese patients with type 2 diabetes treated with metformin. Diabetes Care. 2002;25(7):1123–8.
8. Kelley DE, Bray GA, Pi-Sunyer FX, et al. Clinical efficacy of orlistat therapy in overweight and obese patients with insulin-treated type 2 diabetes: a 1-year randomized controlled trial. Diabetes Care. 2002;25(6):1033–41.
9. Halpern A, Mancini MC, Suplicy H, et al. Latin-American trial of orlistat for weight loss and improvement in glycaemic profile in obese diabetic patients. Diabetes Obes Metab. 2003;5(3):180–8.
10. Chanoine J-P, Hauptman J, Boldrin M, et al. Beneficial effects on orlistat on weight and body composition in obese adolescents [abstract no. T7b:P7b-030 plus poster]. Int J Obes. 2004;28(Suppl. 1):S195.
11. Rossner S, Sjostrom L, Noack R, et al. Weight loss, weight maintenance, and improved cardiovascular risk factors after 2 years treatment with orlistat for obesity: European Orlistat Obesity Study Group. Obes Res. 2000;8(1):49–61.
12. Broom I, Lindgarde F, Guy-Grand B, et al. Weight loss at lead-in is not a predictor for weight loss success with orlistat in patients with multimorbidities. Int J Obes. 2004;28Suppl. 1:S152.
13. Rissanen A, Lean M, Rossner S, et al. Predictive value of early weight loss in obesity management with orlistat: an evidence-based assessment of prescribing guidelines. Int J Obes Relat Metab Disord. 2003;27(1):103–9.
14. Lucas CP, Boldrin MN, Reaven GM. Effect of orlistat added to diet (30% of calories from fat) on plasma lipids, glucose, and insulin in obese patients with hypercholesterolemia. Am J Cardiol. 2003;91(8):961–4.
15. Bloch KV, Salles GF, Muxfeldt ES, et al. Orlistat in hypertensive overweight/obese patients: results of a randomized clinical trial. J Hypertens. 2003;21(11):2159–65.
16. Torgerson JS, Hauptman J, Boldrin M, et al. Efficacy of orlistat plus lifestyle changes in risk reduction of type 2 diabetes in obese patients with metabolic syndrome: a comparative analysis using National Cholesterol Education Program Adult Treatment Panel III vs European group for the study of insulin resistance criteria [abstract no. 690]. Diabetologia. 2004;47(Suppl. 1):A249.
17. Jacob S, Ziegler O, Toplak H, et al. Orlistat improves all components of the metabolic syndrome in overweight and obese patients on two diets [abstract no. T5P5b-011 plus poster presented at the 13th European Congress on Obesity; 2004 May 26–9; Prague]. Int J Obes. 2004;28(Suppl. 1):S154.
18. Lamotte M, Annemans L, Lefever A, et al. A health economic model to assess the long-term effects and cost-effectiveness of orlistat in obese type 2 diabetic patients. Diabetes Care. 2002;25(2):303–8.
19. Maetzel A, Ruof J, Covington M, et al. Economic evaluation of orlistat in overweight and obese patients with type 2 diabetes mellitus. Pharmacoeconomics. 2003;21(7):501–12.
20. Broom I, Hughes E, Dodson P, et al. The role of orlistat in the treatment of obese patients with mild to moderate hypercholesterolaemia: consequences for coronary risk. Br J Cardiol. 2002;9(8):460–8.
21. Lindgarde F. The effect of orlistat on body weight and coronary heart disease risk profile in obese patients: the Swedish Multimorbidity Study. J Intern Med. 2000;248(3):245–54.

22. Finer N, James WP, Kopelman PG, et al. One-year treatment of obesity: a randomized, double-blind, placebo-controlled, multicentre study of orlistat, a gastrointestinal lipase inhibitor. Int J Obes Relat Metab Disord. 2000;24(3):306–13.
23. Hill JO, Hauptman J, Anderson JW. Orlistat, a lipase inhibitor, for weight maintenance after conventional dieting: a 1-year study. Am J Clin Nutr. 1999;69:1108–16.
24. McDuffie JR, Calis KA, Uwaifo GI, et al. Three-month tolerability of orlistat in adolescents with obesity-related comorbid conditions. Obes Res. 2002;10(7):642–50.
25. Zhi J, Moore R, Kanitra L. The effect of short-term (21-day) orlistat treatment on the physiologic balance of six selected macrominerals and microminerals in obese adolescents. J Am Coll Nutr. 2003;22(5):357–62.
26. Hollander PA, Elbein SC, Hirsch IB, et al. Role of orlistat in the treatment of obese patients with type 2 diabetes: a 1-year randomized double-blind study. Diabetes Care. 1998;21(8):1288–94.
27. Davidson MH, Hauptman J, DiGirolamo M, et al. Weight control and risk factor reduction in obese subjects treated for 2 years with orlistat: a randomized controlled trial. JAMA. 1999;281(3):235–42.
28. Guerciolini R. Mode of action of orlistat. Int J Obes Relat Metab Disord. 1997;21(Suppl 3):S12–23.
29. Shick SM, Wing RR, Klem ML, McGuire MT, Hill JO, Seagle H. Persons successful at long-term weight loss and maintenance continue to consume a low-energy, low-fat diet. J Am Diet Assoc. 1998;89:408–13.
30. McGuire MT, Wing RR, Klem ML, Hill JO. Behavioural strategies of individuals who have maintained long-term weight losses. Obes Res. 1999;7:334–41.
31. McGuire MT, Wing RR, Klem ML, Lang W, Hill JO. What predicts weight regain in a group of successful weight losers? J Consult Clin Psychol. 1999;67:177–85.
32. Wing RR, Hill JO. Successful weight loss maintenance. Annu Rev Nutr. 2001;21:232–341.
33. Okauchi Y, Nishizawa H, Funahashi T, et al. Reduction of visceral fat is associated with decrease in the number of metabolic risk in Japanese men. Diabetes Care. 2007;30:2392–4.
34. Look AHEAD Research group, Pi-Sunyer X, Blackburn G, et al. Reduction in weight and cardiovascular disease risk factors in individuals with type 2 diabetes: one-year results of the look AHEAD trial. Diabetes Care. 2007;30:1374–83.
35. Hiuge-Shimizu A, Kishida K, Funahashi T, et al. Absolute value of visceral fat area measured on computed tomography scans and obesity-related cardiovascular risk factors in large-scale Japanese general population (the VACATION-J study). Ann Med. 2012;44:82–92.
36. Goldstein DJ, Parvin JH. Long-term weight loss: the effect of pharmacologic agents. Am J Clin Nutr. 1994;60:647–57.
37. A Report by the Royal College of Physicians. Clinical management of overweight and obese patients with particular reference to the use of drugs. London: Royal College of Physicians; 1998.
38. Kolanowski J. A risk–benefit assessment of anti-obesity drugs. Drug Safety. 1999;20:119–31.
39. Scheen AJ, Lefèbvre PJ. Pharmacological treatment of obesity: present status. Int J Obes Relat Metab Disord. 1999;23: (Suppl 1):S47–53.
40. Hill JO, Hauptman J, Anderson JW, Fujioka K, O'Neil PM, Smith DK, Zavoral JH, Aronne LJ. Orlistat, a lipase inhibitor, for weight maintenance after conventional dieting: a 1-y study. Am J Clin Nutr. 1999;69:1108–16.
41. Zavoral JH. Treatment with orlistat reduces cardiovascular risk in obese patients. J Hypertens. 1998;16:2013–7.
42. Hecker KD, Kris-Etherton PM, Zhao G, Coval S, Jeor SS. Impact of body weight and weight loss on cardiovascular risk factors. Curr Atheroscler Rep. 1999;1:236–42.
43. Van Gaal LF, Wauters MA, De Leeuw IH. The beneficial effects of modest weight loss on cardiovascular risk factors. Int J Obes Relat Metab Disord. 1997;21(Suppl 1):S5–9.

44. Muls E, Kempen K, Vansant G, Cobbaert C, Saris W. The effects of weight loss and apoprotein E polymorphism on serum lipids, apolipoproteins A-I and B, and lipoprotein(a). Int J Obes Relat Metab Disord. 1993;17:711–6.
45. Woo KS, Donnan SPB. Epidemiology of coronary arterial disease in the Chinese. Intern J Card. 1989;24:83–93. https://doi.org/10.1016/0167-5273(89)90045-4.
46. Janus ED, Postiglione A, Singh RB, Lewis B. The modernization of Asia: implications for coronary heart disease. Circulation. 1996;94:2671–3.
47. Montaye M, De Bacquer D, De Backer G, Amouyel P. Overweight and obesity: a major challenge for coronary heart disease secondary prevention in clinical practice in Europe. Eur Heart J. 2000;21:808–13. https://doi.org/10.1053/euhj.1999.1854.
48. Hutton B, Fergusson D. Changes in body weight and serum lipid profile in obese patients treated with orlistat in addition to a hypocaloric diet: a systemic review of randomized clinical trials. Am J Clin Nutr. 2004;80:1461–8.
49. European Agency for the Evaluation of Medicinal Products. Committee for Proprietary Medicinal Products European Public Assessment Report (EPAR): Xenical. London: EMEA; 1998. Available from: http://www.eudra.org/humandocs/humans/epar/xenical/xenical.htm
50. Lean MEJ. Is long-term weight loss possible? Br J Nutr. 2000;83(Suppl 1):S103–11.
51. National Institute for Clinical Excellence. Orlistat for the treatment of obesity in adults. Available from: http://www.nice.org.uk/pdf/orlistatguidance.pdf; 2001.
52. National Institutes of Health. Clinical guidelines on the identification, evaluation, and treatment of overweight and obesity in adults—the evidence report. Obes Res. 1998;6:51S–209S.
53. Brochu M, Tchernof A, Turner AN, Ades PA, Poehlman ET. Is there a threshold of visceral fat loss that improves the metabolic profile in obese postmenopausal women? Metabolism. 2003;52:599–604.
54. Anderson J, Schwartz S, Hauptman J, Boldrin M, Bansal V, Hale C. Low-dose orlistat effects on body weight of mildly to moderately overweight individuals: a 16 week, double-blind, placebo controlled trial. Ann Pharmacother. 2006;40:1717–23.
55. Anderson JW. Orlistat for the management of overweight individuals and obesity: a review of potential for the 60 mg, over-the-counter dosage. Expert Opin Pharmacother. 2007;8:1733–42.
56. Schwartz SM, Bansal VP, Hale C, Rossi M, Engle JP. Compliance, behavior change, and weight loss with orlistat in an over-the-counter setting. Obesity. 2008;16:623–9.
57. Kelley DE, Kuller LH, McKolanis TM, Harper P, Mancino J, Kalhan S. Effects of moderate weight loss and orlistat on insulin resistance, regional adiposity, and fatty acids in type 2 diabetes. Diabetes Care. 2004;27:33–40.
58. Tiikkainen M, Bergholm R, Rissanen A, Aro A, Salminen I, Tamminen M, et al. Effects of equal weight loss with orlistat and placebo on body fat and serum fatty acid composition and insulin resistance in obese women. Am J Clin Nutr. 2004;79:22–30.
59. Chanoine JP, Hampl S, Jensen C, Boldrin M, Hauptman J. Effect of orlistat on weight and body composition in obese adolescents: a randomized controlled trial. JAMA. 2005;293:2873–83.
60. Dixon JB, Strauss BJ, Laurie C, O'Brien PE. Changes in body composition with weight loss: obese subjects randomized to surgical and medical programs. Obesity. 2007;15:1187–98.
61. Thomas EL, Brynes AE, McCarthy J, Goldstone AP, Hajnal JV, Saeed N, et al. Preferential loss of visceral fat following aerobic exercise, measured by magnetic resonance imaging. Lipids. 2000;35:769–76.
62. Ross R, Janssen I, Dawson J, Kungl AM, Kuk JL, Wong SL, et al. Exercise-induced reduction in obesity and insulin resistance in women: a randomized controlled trial. Obes Res. 2004;12:789–98.
63. Styne MD. Childhood and adolescent obesity. Prevalence and significance. Pediatr Clin North Am. 2001;48:823–54.
64. Orlistat: a second look. At best, a minor adjunct to dietary measures. Prescribe Int. 2002;11:10–2.
65. Hirosawa K, Fukami T, Nakano M, Nakajima M. Evaluation of drug-drug interactions via inhibition of hydrolases by orlistat, an anti-obesity drug. Drug Metab Dispos. 2023;

66. Zhao G, Zhang Q, Wu F, Yin S, Xie Y, Liu H. Comparison of weight loss and adverse events of obesity drugs in children and adolescents: a systematic review and meta-analysis. Expert Rev Clin Pharmacol. 2022:1–7.
67. Yu CC, Li AM, Chan KO, Chook P, Kam JT, Au CT, So RC, Sung RY, McManus AM. Orlistat improves endothelial function in obese adolescents: a randomised trial. J Paediatr Child Health. 2013;49(11):969–75.
68. Maahs D, de Serna DG, Kolotkin RL, Ralston S, Sandate J, Qualls C, Schade DS. Randomized, double-blind, placebo-controlled trial of orlistat for weight loss in adolescents. Endocr Pract. 2006;12(1):18–28.
69. Norgren S, Danielsson P, Jurold R, Lötborn M, Marcus C. Orlistat treatment in obese prepubertal children: a pilot study. Acta Paediatr. 2003;92(6):666–70.
70. Li Z, Maglione M, Tu W, Mojica W, Arterburn D, Shugarman LR, et al. Meta-analysis: pharmacologic treatment of obesity. Ann Intern Med. 2005;142:532–46.
71. Chilton M, Dunkley A, Carter P, Davies M, Khunti K, Gray L. The effect of antiobesity drugs on waist circumference: a mixed treatment comparison. Diabetes Obes Metabolism. 2014;16(3):237–47.
72. Williamson D, Pamuk E, Thun M, et al. Prospective study of intentional weight loss and mortality in never-smoking overweight US white women aged 40–64 years. Am J Epidemiol. 1995;141:1128–41.
73. Jung RT. Obesity as a disease. Br Med Bull. 1997;53:307–21.
74. Zhang Y, Proenca R, Maffei M, et al. Positional cloning of the mouse obese gene and its human homologue. Nature. 1994;372:425–32.
75. Batterham RL, le Roux CW, Cohen MA, et al. Pancreatic polypeptide reduces appetite and food intake in humans. J Clin Endocrinol Metab. 2003;88:3989–92.
76. Schwartz MW, Woods SC, Porte D Jr, et al. Central nervous system control of food intake. Nature. 2000;404:661–71.
77. Sumithran P, Prendergast LA, Delbridge E, et al. Long-term persistence of hormonal adaptations to weight loss. N Engl J Med. 2011;365:1597–604.
78. Rosenbaum M, Hirsch J, Gallagher DA, et al. Long-term persistence of adaptive thermogenesis in subjects who have maintained a reduced body weight. Am J Clin Nutr. 2008;88:906–12.
79. Hogan S, Fleury A, Hadvary P, et al. Studies on the antiobesity activity of tetrahydrolipstatin, a potent and selective inhibitor of pancreatic lipase. Int J Obes. 1987;11(Suppl 3):35–42.
80. Hauptman J, Jeunet F, Hartmann D. Initial studies in humans with the novel gastrointestinal lipase inhibitor Ro 18-0647 (tetrahydrolipstatin). Am J Clin Nutr. 1992;55(Suppl):309S–13S.
81. Zhi J, Melia A, Guerciolini R, et al. Retrospective population-based analysis of the dose-response (fecal fat excretion) relationship of orlistat in normal and obese volunteers. Clin Pharmacol Ther. 1994;56:82–5.
82. Jacob S, Rabbia M, Meier M, et al. Orlistat 120 mg improves glycaemic control in type 2 diabetic patients with or without concurrent weight loss. Diabetes Obes Metab. 2009;11:361–71.
83. Fabricatore A, Wadden T, Moore R, et al. Attrition from randomized controlled trials of pharmacological weight loss agents: a systematic review and analysis. Obes Rev. 2009;10:333–41.
84. Sjöstrom L, Rissanen A, Andersen T, et al. Randomised placebo-controlled trial of orlistat for weight loss and prevention of weight regain in obese patients. Lancet. 1998;352:167–73.
85. Davidson M, Hauptman J, DiGirolamo M, et al. Weight control and risk factor reduction in obese subjects treated for 2 years with orlistat. JAMA. 1999;281:235–42.
86. Hauptman J, Lucas C, Boldrin M, et al. Orlistat in the long-term treatment of obesity in primary care settings. Arch Fam Med. 2000;9:160–7.
87. Padwal R, Rucker D, Li S, et al. Long-term pharmacotherapy for obesity and overweight (review). Cochrane Database Syst Rev. 2003:CD004094.
88. Smith S, Stenlof K, Greenway F, et al. Orlistat 60 mg reduces visceral adipose tissue: a 24-week randomized, placebo-controlled, multicentre trial. Obesity. 2011;19:1796–803.
89. Yanovski S, Yanovski J. Long-term drug treatment for obesity: a systematic and clinical review. JAMA. 2014;311:74–86.

90. Royal College of Physicians Working Party. Overweight and Obese Patients: Principles of Management with Particular Reference to the Use of Drugs. London: The Royal College of Physicians; 1997.
91. Fricker J. Balancing the risks of anti-obesity pills. Lancet. 1997;349:1374.
92. Roche Products Limited. Orlistat, Summary of Product Characteristics. August 1998.
93. Stephens MDB (ed). Introduction. Detection of new adverse drug reactions. 3rd ed. Great Britain: Macmillan Publishers Ltd; 1992. p. 17.
94. Stephens MDB (ed). Sample size considerations for pharmacoepidemiology studies. In: Pharmacoepidemiology. 2nd ed. John Wiley & Sons Ltd: UK; 1994. p. 29–38.
95. James WPT, Avenell A, Broom J, Whitehead J. A one year trial to assess the value of orlistat in the management of obesity. Int J Obes Relat Metab Disord. 1997;21(Suppl 3):S24–30.
96. Drent ML, Larsson I, William-Olsson T, Quaade F, Czubayko F, von Bergmann K, Strobel W, Sjöström L, van der Veen EA. Orlistat, a lipase inhibitor, in the treatment of human obesity: a multiple dose study. Int J Obes Relat Metab Disord. 1995;19:221–6.
97. Bray GA, Greenway FL. Current and potential drugs for treatment of obesity. Endocrine Reviews. 1999;20:805–75.
98. Vahouny GV, Krutchevsky M, editors. Dietary fiber: basic and clinical aspects. New York: Plenum Press; 1986. p. 181–209.
99. Wilmink T, Frick TW. Drug-induced pancreatitis. Drug Safety. 1996;14(6):406–23.
100. Canadian Adverse Drug Reaction Newsletter. 2000, 10 (2): http://www.hc-sc.gc.ca/dhp-mps/alt_formats/hpfb-dgpsa/pdf/medeff/carn-bcei_v10n2_e.pdf
101. Tothill P, Avenell A, Reid DM. Precision and accuracy of measurements of whole-body bone mineral: comparison between Hologic, Lunar and Norland dual-energy x-ray absorptiometers. Br J Radiol. 1994;67:1210–7.
102. Tothill R, Avenell A, Love J, Reid DM. Comparisons between Hologic, Lunar and Norland dual-energy x-ray absorptiometers and other techniques used for whole-body soft tissue measurements. Eur J Clin Nutr. 1994;48:781–94.
103. Gotfredsen A, Bæksgaard L, Hilsted J. Body composition analysis by DEXA by using dynamically changing samarium filtration. J Appl Physiol. 1997;82:1200–9.
104. Hendel HW, Gotfredsen A, Andersen T, Højgaard L, Hilsted J. Body composition during weight loss in obese patients estimated by dual energy x-ray absorptiometry and by total body potassium. Int J Obes Relat Disord. 1996;20:1111–9.
105. Mosekilde L, Charles P, Lindegreen P. Determinants for serum 1,25-dihydroxycholecalciferol in primary hyperparathyroidism. Bone Miner. 1989;5:279–90.
106. Lund B, Sorensen OH. Measurement of 25-hydroxyvitamin D in serum and its relation to sunshine, age and vitamin D intake in the Danish population. Scand J Clin Lab Invest. 1979;39:23–30.
107. Hyldstrup L et al. Presented at the IXth International Conference on Calcium Regulating Hormones and Bone Metabolism Nice 1986.
108. Bertels H, Bohmer M, Heierli C. Serum creatinine dertimination without protein precipitation. Clin Chim Acta. 1972;37:193–7.
109. Rickers H, Balslev I, Foltved H, Rødbro P. Bone mineral content before and after bypass operation in obese patients. Acta Med Scand. 1981;209:203–7.
110. Krølner B, Ranløv PJ, Clemmesen T, Nielsen PS. Bone loss after gastroplasty for morbid obesity: side-effect or adaptive response to weight reduction? Lancet. 1982;i:956–7.
111. Danø P, Christiansen C. Calcium absorption and bone mineral content following intestinal shunt operation in obesity. Scand J Gastroenterol. 1974;9:775–9.
112. Hey H, Lund B, Sørensen OH, Lund BJ, Christensen MS. Impairment of vitamin D and bone metabolism in patients with bypass operation for obesity. Acta Med Scand. 1979;624(Suppl):73–8.
113. Compston JE, Vedi S, Gianetta E, Watson G, Civalleri D, Scopinaro N. Bone histomorphometry and vitamin D status after biliopancreatic bypass for obesity. Gastroenterology. 1984;87:350–6.

114. Field AE, Coakley EA, Must A, et al. Impact of overweight on the risk of developing common chronic diseases during a 10-year period. Arch Intern Med. 2001;161(13):1581–6.
115. Brandle M, Honghong Z, Smith B, et al. The direct medical cost of type 2 diabetes. Diabetes Care. 2003;26:2300–4.
116. Foxcroft DR, Milne R. Orlistat for the treatment of obesity: rapid review and cost-effectiveness model. Obes Rev. 2000;1:121–6.
117. LFN. Decision to reimburse orlistat in Sweden for diabetic obese patients and obese patients with a BMI>35. Läkemedelsförmånsnämnden; 2003.
118. Curran MP, Scott LJ. Spotlight on orlistat in the management of patients with obesity. Treatments in Endocrinology; 2005. https://doi.org/10.2165/00024677-200504020-00006.
119. Krempf M, Louvet J-P, Allanic H, Miloradovich T, Joubert J-M, Attali J-R. Weight reduction and long-term maintenance after 18 months treatment with orlistat for obesity. Int J Obesity. 2003; https://doi.org/10.1038/sj.ijo.0802281.
120. Shirai K, Tanaka M, Fujita T, Fujii Y, Shimomasuda M, Sakai S, Samukawa Y. Reduction of excessive visceral fat and safety with 52-week administration of lipase inhibitor orlistat in japanese: long-term clinical study. Adv Therap. 2018; https://doi.org/10.1007/s12325-018-0822-x.
121. Muls E, Kolanowski J, Scheen A, Van Gaal L. The effects of orlistat on weight and on serum lipids in obese patients with hypercholesterolemia: a randomized, double-blind, placebo-controlled, multicentre study. Int J Obesity. 2001; https://doi.org/10.1038/sj.ijo.0801814.
122. Chan KW, Leung WS, Fung YS, Hung HF, Tsui P, Chu H, Chan YW, Ko GTC, Yeung VTF. The effects of diet and orlistat on body weight and lipid profiles in high risk Chinese patients with coronary artery disease, obesity and hypercholesterolemia. Irish J Med Sci. 2009; https://doi.org/10.1007/s11845-009-0291-y.
123. Rissanen A, Lean M, Rössner S, Segal KR, Sjöström L. Predictive value of early weight loss in obesity management with orlistat: an evidence-based assessment of prescribing guidelines. In J Obesity. 2003; https://doi.org/10.1038/sj.ijo.0802165.
124. Thomas EL, Makwana A, Newbould R, Rao AW, Gambarota G, Frost G, Delafont B, Mishra RG, Matthews PM, Berk ES, Schwartz SM, Bell JD, Beaver JD. Pragmatic study of orlistat 60 mg on abdominal obesity. Eur J Clin Nutr. 2011; https://doi.org/10.1038/ejcn.2011.108
125. Ozkan B, Bereket A, Turan S, Keskin S. Addition of orlistat to conventional treatment in adolescents with severe obesity. Eur J Pediatr. 2004; https://doi.org/10.1007/s00431-004-1534-6.
126. Nikniaz Z, Nikniaz L, Farhangi MA, Mehralizadeh H, Salekzamani S. Effect of Orlistat on anthropometrics and metabolic indices in children and adolescents: a systematic review and meta-analysis. BMC Endocrine Disorders. 2023; https://doi.org/10.1186/s12902-023-01390-7.
127. Sumithran P, Proietto J. Benefit-risk assessment of orlistat in the treatment of obesity. Drug Safety. 2014; https://doi.org/10.1007/s40264-014-0210-7.
128. Acharya NV, Wilton LV, Shakir SAW. Safety profile of orlistat: results of a prescription-event monitoring study. Int J Obesity. 2006; https://doi.org/10.1038/sj.ijo.0803323.
129. Cavaliere H, Floriano I, Medeiros-Neto G. Gastrointestinal side effects of orlistat may be prevented by concomitant prescription of natural fibers (psyllium mucilloid). Int J Obesity. 2001; https://doi.org/10.1038/sj.ijo.0801645.
130. Napier S, Thomas M. 36 year old man presenting with pancreatitis and a history of recent commencement of orlistat case report. Nutr J. 2006; https://doi.org/10.1186/1475-2891-5-19.
131. Gotfredsen A, Westergren Hendel H, Andersen T. Influence of orlistat on bone turnover and body composition. Int J Obesity. 2001; https://doi.org/10.1038/sj.ijo.0801639.
132. Hertzman P. The cost effectiveness of orlistat in a 1-year weight-management programme for treating overweight and obese patients in Sweden. PharmacoEconomics. 2005; https://doi.org/10.2165/00019053-200523100-00004.

Chapter 3
Fixed Combination Anti-obesity Medications

Shilpa Chugh Garcha and Sanjay Kalra

Two combination drug therapies phentermine/topiramate ER and naltrexone ER/bupropion ER have been approved by USFDA for long term management of obesity.

Phentermine/topiramate ER combination therapy

Phentermine/topiramate ER is the first combination drug approved for long-term use in the management of obesity.

Phentermine, a sympathomimetic drug, as a single agent has been approved for short-term use for weight loss. Topiramate, the other drug in this combination is an anti-epileptic agent and is a gamma-aminobutyric acid (GABA) receptor agonist, glutamate antagonist, and inhibitor of carbonic anhydrase.

As per one of the studies, included in this chapter, topiramate has been studied in obese individuals for its effect on food intake and preferences, satiety, and resting metabolic rate. Topiramate-induced weight loss is seen mainly due to reduced energy intake rather than energy expenditure. However, topiramate has not been approved as a single agent for the treatment of obesity.

The efficacy of phentermine/topiramate ER has been studied to confirm its long-term safety and efficacy in many clinical trials including EQUATE, EQUIP, CONQUER, and in the SEQUEL extension.

Phentermine/topiramate ER combination mainly causes weight loss by decreasing appetite and increasing satiety. The use of this combination has been shown to reduce body weight, improve cardiovascular risk factors, lower the incidence of type 2 diabetes, and have the potential to impact health outcomes.

Phentermine/topiramate ER combination is approved for chronic weight management along with reduced-calorie diet and increased physical activity in adults with body mass index (BMI) of $\geq$30 kg/m^2 (obese) or $\geq$27 kg/m^2 (overweight) in the

S. C. Garcha (✉)
Sonepat, Haryana, India

S. Kalra
Department of Endocrinology, Bharti Hospital, Karnal, Haryana, India

S. C. Garcha, S. Kalra (eds.), *Drugs for Medical Management of Obesity*,
https://doi.org/10.1007/978-981-96-1651-0_3

presence of at least one weight-related comorbidity such as hypertension, type 2 diabetes mellitus, or dyslipidemia. In the year 2022, the FDA approved the use of phentermine/topiramate ER in children ≥12 years of age [1].

One of the studies discusses the use of phentermine/topiramate ER in the paediatric population. The studies conducted on adolescents indicate a significant lowering of BMI in adolescents when used along with lifestyle modifications. However, there have been concerns about changes in bone mineral density on long-term use. There is a need for more studies to explore long-term health outcomes with the use of phentermine/topiramate combination in adolescents.

We have included a case report that explores the off-label use of phentermine/topiramate ER in a patient with obesity and sleep-related eating disorder (SRED), where in patient's nocturnal binge eating episodes stopped. Hence, the authors identified it's use as off-label in the management of SRED.

One of the studies talk about its preclinical development for patients with non-alcoholic steatohepatitis (NASH) and clinical development for sleep apnea syndrome and type 2 diabetes in obese patients.

Many studies have also explored the impact of weight loss by phentermine/topiramate ER on the quality of life (QoL) of patients and its cost-effectiveness. One of the studies utilized the data of CONQUER trial and evaluated the incremental cost-effectiveness ratio (ICER) of phentermine/topiramate ER from a payer perspective wherein the ICER was favourable and QoL benefits persisted after stopping the treatment. Another study explored its impact on improving health-related quality of life (HRQOL) and highlighted that there are other associated factors as well that can impact the QoL such as depressive symptoms, physical activity, and social support.

Naltrexone ER/bupropion ER combination therapy

In 2014, FDA approved the combination of naltrexone, a μ-opioid receptor antagonist, and bupropion, a dopamine and norepinephrine reuptake inhibitor for long-term use in patients with obesity [2].

Oral naltrexone extended-release/bupropion extended-release (naltrexone ER/bupropion ER) is recommended as an adjunct to a reduced-calorie diet and increased physical activity for chronic weight management in adults with an initial BMI of ≥30 kg/m^2 (obese), or ≥27 kg/m^2 (overweight) in the presence of at least one weight-related co-morbidity (such as hypertension, type 2 diabetes, or dyslipidemia) [2].

Many studies have explored the mechanism of action, efficacy, and safety of this drug combination. One of the studies included in this chapter highlights the neural targets of these medications; the hypothalamic melanocortin system, mesolimbic dopamine circuit, and the brain's reward pathways which further affect food intake and cravings. These studies underscore the effectiveness of this drug combination in reducing body weight as compared to placebo and causing notable improvements in cardiometabolic parameters, quality of life, and control over eating.

One of the studies explores the efficacy and safety of naltrexone ER/bupropion ER in the management of altered eating behaviours and weight loss in binge eating disorder (BED). The study noticed the efficacy and tolerability of naltrexone ER/bupropion ER along with a reduced-calorie diet and increased physical activity in improving pathological eating behaviour and losing weight in obese patients with BED.

Many centrally-acting drugs for the management of obesity have been associated with psychiatric adverse events (PAEs). A post hoc analysis of the data pooled from placebo-controlled clinical trials was done in one of the studies and it focused on the psychiatric safety profile of naltrexone ER/bupropion ER. It was seen that anxiety and sleep disorder-related PAEs were more frequent with naltrexone ER/bupropion ER, however, depression-related adverse events were less common with naltrexone ER/bupropion ER as compared to placebo. This study underscores the importance of investigating its effects on individuals with existing depression or those taking antidepressants.

Also, there has been interest in the use of these drug combinations along with other concomitant medications as a post-hoc analysis of the LIGHT trial explored the concomitant use of naltrexone ER/bupropion ER with incretin agents such as dipeptidyl peptidase-4 inhibitors (DPP-4) and glucagon-like peptide-1 receptor agonists (GLP-1 RAs). The study suggested that naltrexone ER/bupropion ER is an effective and well-tolerated option for weight loss among type 2 diabetes patients taking incretin therapies.

The efficacy of these drug combinations is well-established in the management of obesity. Looking forward more studies are needed to evaluate the role of these combination therapies in eating disorders associated with obesity and continuous monitoring of the patients is advisable for any psychiatric adverse effects. Despite increasing concern for economic implications associated with obesity, cost-effectiveness studies are lacking, so, health economic studies should be an area of future research.

References for Introduction

(1) QSYMIA (phentermine and topiramate extended-release capsules). U.S. Food and Drug Administration website. https://www.accessdata.fda.gov/drugsatfda_docs/label/2023/022580s023lbl.pdf Revised June 2023. Accessed 19 Oct 2024
(2) CONTRAVE (naltrexone HCl and bupropion HCl) Extended Release Tablets. U.S. Food and Drug Administration website. https://www.accessdata.fda.gov/drugsatfda_docs/label/2014/200063s000lbl.pdf Revised Sep 2014. Accessed 8 Aug 2024

3.1 Machine Generated Summaries

Disclaimer: The summaries in this chapter were generated from Springer Nature publications using abstractive AI auto-summarization: An abstraction-based summarizer creates new text based on deep learning. New phrases are created to summarize the content. As the constituted sentences are machine selected, they may not fully reflect the body of the work, so we strongly advise that the original content is read and cited. The auto-generated summaries were curated by the editor to meet Springer Nature publication standards.

Machine generated keywords: phentermine-topiramate, topiramate, naltrexone, chronic weight, reducedcalorie diet.

The Effect of Topiramate on Energy Balance in Obese Men: A 6-Month Double-Blind Randomized Placebo-Controlled Study with a 6-Month Open-Label Extension [72]

This is a machine-generated summary of:

Tremblay, Angelo; Chaput, Jean-Philippe; Bérubé-Parent, Sonia; Prud'homme, Denis; Leblanc, Claude; Alméras, Natalie; Després, Jean-Pierre: The effect of topiramate on energy balance in obese men: a 6-month double-blind randomized placebo-controlled study with a 6-month open-label extension [72]

Published in: European Journal of Clinical Pharmacology (2007)

Link to original: https://doi.org/10.1007/s00228-006-0220-1

If you want to cite the papers, please refer to the original.

For technical reasons we could not place the page where the original quote is coming from.

Research highlights

Introduction:

Obesity, a complex and multifaceted condition, continues to challenge the medical community, necessitating the development of new pharmacological interventions. Current long-term treatments like sibutramine have limitations and side effects that underscore the need for alternative therapies. Topiramate (TPM), an antiepileptic drug, has emerged as a potential weight loss agent due to its observed "side effect" of reducing body weight. Despite this, the mechanisms by which TPM affects energy balance remain unclear. Now a new study by Angelo Tremblay and colleagues seeks to bridge this knowledge gap by exploring TPM's impact on food preferences, satiety, food intake, resting metabolic rate (RMR), and 24-hour energy expenditure in obese individuals.

Main Body:

Tremblay et al.'s research is grounded in rigorous methodology, employing a 6-month randomized, double-blind, placebo-controlled trial with an additional open-label extension. The study meticulously selected non-smoking, sedentary men with abdominal obesity, dyslipidemia, and body mass index (BMI) $\geq$27 and $\leq$40 kg/m^2 to participate. Participants were randomized to receive either TPM or placebo and were monitored through various stages including a 24-hour energy expenditure substudy. The researchers employed a comprehensive approach to measure changes in body composition and metabolic rates using standardized breakfasts, buffet-type meals for assessing food intake preferences, and indirect calorimetry for RMR.

The study's findings are compelling; TPM significantly reduced appetite and altered energy utilization efficiency through mechanisms such as increased lipoprotein lipase activity and uncoupling protein expression. These changes were not merely transient; weight loss continued over the year-long study period with TPM being generally well-tolerated by participants.

Conclusion:

The advances made by Tremblay et al.'s study are noteworthy; they demonstrate that TPM can significantly reduce body weight in obese patients without compromising satiety levels. The weight loss associated with TPM is primarily due to a reduction in energy intake rather than an increase in energy expenditure. This insight into the drug's mechanism of action could pave the way for future obesity treatments that target similar pathways. As Tremblay notes, "TPM has a significant effect on systems involved in the regulation of energy balance," suggesting that it could be a valuable tool in managing obesity while maintaining patient comfort and satiety—a promising direction for future research and therapeutic strategies.

Phentermine and Topiramate Extended Release (Qsymia™) [73]

This is a machine-generated summary of:

Cameron, Fiona; Whiteside, Glenn; McKeage, Kate: Phentermine and Topiramate Extended Release (Qsymia™) [73]

Published in: Drugs (2012)

Link to original: https://doi.org/10.2165/11640860-000000000-00000

If you want to cite the papers, please refer to the original.

For technical reasons we could not place the page where the original quote is coming from.

Research highlights

Obesity remains a critical challenge in public health, with existing treatments often falling short in providing sustainable weight management. While lifestyle changes and pharmacological interventions are standard, their long-term efficacy is limited. Now a new study by Fiona Cameron and colleagues introduces a promising pharmacological approach: a combination of low-dose phentermine and extended-release topiramate in a once-daily oral capsule designed to maximize weight loss benefits while minimizing side effects.

Three phase III trials were conducted to evaluate the efficacy and safety of this novel combination. The trials—EQUATE, EQUIP, and CONQUER—involved a diverse group of obese adults, some with weight-related comorbidities. Participants underwent a 4-week dose-titration period in all clinical trials. The researchers found that the combination therapy significantly outperformed monotherapies and placebo in reducing body weight, and had positive impact in improving cardiovascular risk factors. Notably, the SEQUEL extension study confirmed the long-term safety and effectiveness of the treatment up to two years.

The study's findings represent a significant advance in obesity pharmacotherapy, offering an effective long-term treatment option for individuals struggling with obesity and its related health issues. The combination therapy's ability to improve quality of life and reduce the incidence of type 2 diabetes underscores its potential impact on patient health outcomes. Further research is going on to explore the broader implications of this treatment for various patient populations, including those with type 2 diabetes or sleep apnoea. The commitment to post-marketing studies will also provide valuable insights into the long-term cardiovascular effects and further studies are planned in specific groups such as pediatric patients.

Phentermine/Topiramate: Pediatric First Approval [74]

This is a machine-generated summary of:

Dhillon, Sohita: Phentermine/Topiramate: Pediatric First Approval [74]

Published in: Pediatric Drugs (2022)

Link to original: https://doi.org/10.1007/s40272-022-00532-z

If you want to cite the papers, please refer to the original.

For technical reasons we could not place the page where the original quote is coming from.

Research highlights

Obesity in adolescents is a critical health issue, with the prevalence among 12- to 19-year-olds in the USA climbing from 15.5% in 1999–2000 to 22.2% in 2017–2020.

Despite lifestyle interventions, many adolescents struggle to manage their weight, leading to the exploration of pharmacotherapies as adjunct treatments. Now a review by Sohita Dhillon explores the efficacy and safety of phentermine/topiramate extended-release capsules for weight management in adolescent obesity.

The review assesses the pharmacokinetics and therapeutic impact of phentermine/topiramate on obese adolescents by including data from randomized, double-blind, placebo-controlled phase 4 study that meticulously evaluated the drug's effects on body mass index (BMI) and safety profile over a 56-week period. Adolescents receiving phentermine/topiramate exhibited consistent drug exposure levels with adults, suggesting similar metabolic processing between the age groups. The study's design also accounted for potential dietary influences by including a reduced-calorie diet and increased physical activity as part of the treatment regimen. The pharmacokinetic properties observed in adolescents were within expected ranges based on adult data.

Findings from various trials are promising, indicating that phentermine/topiramate can significantly reduce BMI in adolescents when combined with lifestyle modifications. The treatment was associated with greater BMI reductions compared to placebo, with some concerns about bone mineral density changes. The review emphasizes the importance of ongoing clinical trials to explore long-term outcomes and additional health benefits.

Phentermine–Topiramate Extended Release for the Dual Treatment of Obesity and Sleep-Related Eating Disorder: A Case Report [75]

This is a machine-generated summary of:

Grunvald, Eduardo; DeConde, Jennifer: Phentermine–topiramate extended release for the dual treatment of obesity and sleep-related eating disorder: a case report [75]

Published in: Journal of Medical Case Reports (2022)

Link to original: https://doi.org/10.1186/s13256-021-03250-1

If you want to cite the papers, please refer to the original.

For technical reasons we could not place the page where the original quote is coming from.

Research highlights

Research Highlight

Obesity is a multifaceted disease influenced by a variety of factors, including eating disorders such as binge eating disorder (BED) and sleep-related eating disorder (SRED), which are often associated with increased body mass index (BMI). Despite the complexity of obesity, pharmacological interventions have shown promise, particularly the combination of phentermine and topiramate extended release (PHEN-TPM ER), approved by the FDA for long-term obesity management. Now a new study by Eduardo Grunvald and Jennifer DeConde presents a case where PHEN-TPM ER not only facilitated weight loss but also resolved pathological hyperphagia at night in a patient with obesity and SRED, underscoring the need for comprehensive screening for eating disorders in obesity treatment.

In this case report, Grunvald and DeConde detail the clinical journey of a male patient with obesity and SRED who was treated with PHEN-TPM ER. The patient's nocturnal eating episodes ceased, and he experienced significant weight loss within two months of treatment. The study meticulously describes the patient's medical history, including unsuccessful weight loss attempts and comorbidities such as fatty liver disease, hypertension, and hypothyroidism. The therapeutic approach combined PHEN-TPM ER with lifestyle modifications, showcasing the medication's dual benefit. The authors emphasize that while PHEN-TPM ER is FDA-approved for obesity treatment, its use in managing SRED represents an off-label application that warrants further investigation.

The main advance highlighted by this study is the potential role of PHEN-TPM ER in treating SRED alongside obesity, suggesting a new avenue for improving patient outcomes. The case demonstrates the importance of recognizing and addressing comorbid eating disorders within obesity management frameworks. As the author notes, "This report demonstrates a potential new tool and will hopefully trigger more research in this area." Looking forward, this case may inspire more research to confirm the efficacy of PHEN-TPM ER in treating SRED and to explore whether this combination could offer even greater benefits for patients struggling with both obesity and nocturnal eating behaviors.

Cost-Effectiveness Analysis of Qsymia for Weight Loss [76]

This is a machine-generated summary of:

Finkelstein, Eric A.; Kruger, Eliza; Karnawat, Sunil: Cost-Effectiveness Analysis of Qsymia for Weight Loss [76]

Published in: PharmacoEconomics (2014)

Link to original: https://doi.org/10.1007/s40273-014-0182-6

If you want to cite the papers, please refer to the original.

For technical reasons we could not place the page where the original quote is coming from.

Research highlights

Background and Knowledge Gap:

Obesity is a critical global health issue, with its prevalence doubling over recent decades and contributing to approximately 2.8 million deaths annually. While obesity's health consequences are well-documented, its economic burden is also profound, with billions spent on related medical expenditures in the United States alone. Despite the known benefits of weight-loss initiatives, current interventions like lifestyle modification and bariatric surgery have limitations in terms of effectiveness and accessibility. Pharmacological treatments have historically been limited due to safety concerns or modest efficacy. Now a new study by Eric A. Finkelstein and colleagues addresses the cost-effectiveness of Qsymia, an FDA-approved drug for chronic weight management, filling a crucial knowledge gap in long-term obesity treatment strategies.

Study Description and Effectiveness:

The study utilized data from the CONQUER trial, a randomized controlled trial assessing Qsymia's effectiveness for weight loss and related comorbidities. Participants included overweight or obese adults with additional risk factors such as elevated blood pressure or cholesterol levels, increased waist circumference or type 2 diabetes managed with lifestyle modification or metformin. The trial demonstrated that Qsymia, combined with diet and exercise, resulted in significant weight loss and improvements in various health parameters compared to placebo. Finkelstein's team extended this analysis by evaluating the incremental cost-effectiveness ratio (ICER) of Qsymia from a payer perspective, considering both direct costs and potential savings from reduced medication use for comorbid conditions.

Advances and Future Directions:

The study's main advance is providing evidence that Qsymia could be a cost-effective treatment option when used alongside diet and exercise for individuals with obesity-related comorbidities. The ICER for Qsymia was favorable under certain conditions, particularly to the extent to which benefits persist after treatment cessation. However, the authors note limitations such as the lack of real-world data on long-term medication adherence and sustained benefits post-treatment. Finkelstein et al.'s work contributes significantly to understanding the economic value of emerging pharmacological interventions in managing obesity.

Health-Related Quality of Life in Two Randomized Controlled Trials of Phentermine/Topiramate for Obesity: What Mediates Improvement? [77]

This is a machine-generated summary of:

Kolotkin, Ronette L.; Gadde, Kishore M.; Peterson, Craig A.; Crosby, Ross D.: Health-related quality of life in two randomized controlled trials of phentermine/topiramate for obesity: What mediates improvement? [77]

Published in: Quality of Life Research (2015)

Link to original: https://doi.org/10.1007/s11136-015-1153-x

If you want to cite the papers, please refer to the original.

For technical reasons we could not place the page where the original quote is coming from.

Research highlights

Introduction:

Obesity and overweight, with their associated health risks, have become a global health challenge. While weight loss is known to improve health-related quality of life (HRQOL), the mechanisms behind these improvements remain unclear. Now a new study by Ronette L. Kolotkin and colleagues delves into the effects of phentermine/topiramate extended-release on HRQOL, exploring whether weight loss is the sole mediator of these benefits or if other factors also contribute.

Main Body:

Kolotkin's team utilized data from the EQUIP and CONQUER trials, focusing on changes in both generic and obesity-specific HRQOL over 56 weeks. They employed mediation analysis to investigate whether variables such as reduction in depressive symptoms or improvement in cardiovascular/glycemic risk markers played a role in enhancing HRQOL. The researchers included patients who completed relevant questionnaires at baseline and week 56, ensuring that temporal precedence was established for mediating variables.

The study's methodology was rigorous, with multiple mediation analyses done to determine if early changes in BMI, depressive symptoms, blood pressure, and HbA1c could mediate later improvements in HRQOL. The authors note that weight loss or BMI reduction was indeed a significant mediator in HRQOL improvements. The research also considered how these mechanisms might vary based on baseline characteristics such as age, gender, race, waist circumference, triglycerides, and history of pain or psychiatric illness.

Conclusion:

Kolotkin's research advances our understanding of how weight loss treatments like phentermine/topiramate improve HRQOL. The study confirms that while BMI reduction is a primary driver of these improvements, other factors like depressive symptoms also play a role. Looking ahead, the author suggests that future research should explore additional mediators such as physical activity and social support to fully grasp the multifaceted relationship between weight management and quality of life. This comprehensive approach could further refine interventions aimed at enhancing the well-being of individuals struggling with obesity.

4-Year Cost Trajectories in Real-World Patients Matched to the Metabolic Profiles of Trial Subjects Before/After Treatment with Phentermine-Topiramate [78]

This is a machine-generated summary of:

Li, James; Reaven, Nancy L.; Funk, Susan E.; McGaughey, Karen; Neovius, Martin: 4-Year Cost Trajectories in Real-World Patients Matched to the Metabolic Profiles of Trial Subjects Before/After Treatment with Phentermine-Topiramate [78]

Published in: Drugs - Real World Outcomes (2015)

Link to original: https://doi.org/10.1007/s40801-015-0021-x

If you want to cite the papers, please refer to the original.

For technical reasons we could not place the page where the original quote is coming from.

Research highlights

Introduction:

Despite public health targets for obesity reduction, the proportion of obese US adults was estimated at 35% in 2012. Obesity is associated with increased all-cause mortality, primarily due to cardiovascular deaths, and multiple comorbidities such as type 2 diabetes mellitus, cardiovascular diseases, and many others. Obese individuals incur higher medical costs, with cost increases of 25% for class I (BMI 30–34.9 kg/m^2) obese individuals and 50% for class II (BMI 35–40 kg/m^2) obese individuals compared with normal weight individuals. Now a new study by James Li and colleagues addresses the economic impact of the anti-obesity drug phentermine-topiramate extended-release (ER), revealing potential cost savings in healthcare utilization.

Methods:

Li's team conducted a retrospective analysis using real-world patient data to estimate changes in medical services and costs associated with metabolic improvements from phentermine-topiramate ER treatment. They matched patients from the CONQUER trial's post- and pre-treatment metabolic profiles to real-world patients over a three-year period, avoiding assumptions about BMI changes. The study focused on both intention-to-treat (ITT) subjects and 'responders'—those who lost ≥5% body weight by the end of the trial. Healthcare utilization was assessed across inpatient, outpatient, emergency department visits, lab tests, and prescriptions.

Results:

The study found that patients matching post-trial CONQUER ITT subjects had fewer outpatient visits and received fewer prescriptions than their pre-trial counterparts, although no significant overall cost difference was observed. However, when focusing on responders, patients matched to post-trial responders had significant savings in outpatient visits, prescription costs, and emergency department visits over three years. These findings suggest that metabolic improvements from phentermine-topiramate ER can lead to reduced healthcare service utilization.

Conclusion:

James Li et al.'s research highlights the potential for anti-obesity treatments like phentermine-topiramate ER to offer economic benefits by reducing healthcare costs associated with obesity-related comorbidities. While no overall cost difference was found in the ITT analysis, responders showed significant savings, indicating that successful weight loss can lead to meaningful reductions in healthcare utilization. Future research should include treatment-related adverse events and compliance costs to provide a more comprehensive understanding of the economic impact of anti-obesity drugs.

Naltrexone ER/Bupropion ER in Obesity Management: A Guide to Its Use [79]

This is a machine-generated summary of:

Greig, Sarah L.; Keating, Gillian M.: Naltrexone ER/bupropion ER in obesity management: a guide to its use [79]

Published in: Drugs & Therapy Perspectives (2015)

Link to original: https://doi.org/10.1007/s40267-015-0253-6

If you want to cite the papers, please refer to the original.

For technical reasons we could not place the page where the original quote is coming from.

Research highlights

Obesity, a chronic disease requiring ongoing management, often proves resistant to traditional interventions like diet, exercise, and behavioral modification. Despite these efforts, many individuals struggle to achieve significant long-term weight loss, highlighting a need for effective pharmacological treatments. Now a new study by Sarah L. Greig and Gillian M. Keating delves into the efficacy and safety of an oral combination drug therapy—naltrexone extended-release (ER)/bupropion ER—designed to complement lifestyle changes for adults with obesity or weight-related comorbidities.

Greig and Keating explores the synergistic effects of naltrexone, a μ-opioid receptor antagonist, and bupropion, a dopamine and norepinephrine reuptake inhibitor. These medications target the hypothalamic melanocortin system and the brain's reward pathways that influence food intake and cravings. This review explored four randomized, placebo-controlled trials (COR-I, -II, BMOD, and Diabetes) where participants also received lifestyle modification advice or underwent intensive behavioral modification programs. The findings indicate that naltrexone ER/bupropion ER significantly reduces body weight compared to placebo, with notable improvements in cardiometabolic parameters and patient-reported outcomes related to quality of life and control over eating.

The main advances highlighted by Greig's study include the clinical efficacy of naltrexone ER/bupropion ER in promoting weight loss and improving various health markers in obese or overweight adults. The research underscores the potential of this pharmacotherapy as an adjunct to lifestyle interventions for chronic weight management. This combination therapy is generally well-tolerated with manageable side effects like nausea, however, further investigation into its long-term cardiovascular impact is planned.

Naltrexone ER/Bupropion ER: A Review in Obesity Management [80]

This is a machine-generated summary of:

Greig, Sarah L.; Keating, Gillian M.: Naltrexone ER/Bupropion ER: A Review in Obesity Management [80]

Published in: Drugs (2015)

Link to original: https://doi.org/10.1007/s40265-015-0427-5

If you want to cite the papers, please refer to the original.

For technical reasons we could not place the page where the original quote is coming from.

Research highlights

Introduction:

The global obesity epidemic has escalated, with rates more than doubling since 1980. This condition elevates the risk of various health issues, including type 2 diabetes, cardiovascular diseases, musculoskeletal disorders, and certain cancers, as well as mortality. Despite lifestyle interventions being the cornerstone of weight management, many individuals fail to achieve sustained weight loss, necessitating additional therapeutic options. Now a new study by Sarah L. Greig and Gillian M. Keating delves into the efficacy and safety of naltrexone extended-release (ER)/ bupropion ER combination therapy for obesity management.

Main Body:

Greig and Keating provides a comprehensive analysis of naltrexone ER/bupropion ER as an adjunct to diet and exercise for chronic weight control in obese or overweight adults with weight-related comorbidities. The study synthesizes data from randomized controlled trials, pharmacodynamic profiles, and pharmacokinetic properties to understand the drug's impact on weight loss and associated health outcomes. The dual-action medication targets both homeostatic and reward pathways in the brain to regulate food intake and body weight. The authors describe how naltrexone ER/bupropion ER works synergistically to regulate food intake and enhance satiety through its effects on the hypothalamic melanocortin system and mesolimbic dopamine circuit.

Conclusion:

The key advancement from Greig and Keating's study is the demonstration of significant weight reduction and improvement in cardiometabolic risk factors with naltrexone ER/bupropion ER therapy compared to placebo. The findings suggest that this pharmacotherapy could fill a critical gap for patients who do not respond adequately to lifestyle modifications alone. Further research is needed to understand the long-term impacts of naltrexone ER/bupropion ER on weight management and cardiovascular health.

An Open-Label Trial on the Efficacy and Tolerability of Naltrexone/ Bupropion SR for Treating Altered Eating Behaviours and Weight Loss in Binge Eating Disorder [81]

This is a machine-generated summary of:

Carbone, Elvira Anna; Caroleo, Mariarita; Rania, Marianna; Calabrò, Giuseppina; Staltari, Filippo Antonio; de Filippis, Renato; Aloi, Matteo; Condoleo, Francesca; Arturi, Franco; Segura-Garcia, Cristina: An open-label trial on the efficacy and tolerability of naltrexone/bupropion SR for treating altered eating behaviours and weight loss in binge eating disorder [81]

Published in: Eating and Weight Disorders - Studies on Anorexia, Bulimia and Obesity (2020)
Link to original: https://doi.org/10.1007/s40519-020-00910-x

If you want to cite the papers, please refer to the original.

For technical reasons we could not place the page where the original quote is coming from.

Research highlights

Introduction:

Binge eating disorder (BED) is the most common eating disorder, affecting individuals across all demographics and contributing to various psychiatric and medical comorbidities, notably obesity. While treatments such as psychotherapy, educational interventions, and pharmacological therapies have been explored, their long-term efficacy remains unproven. Now a new study by Elvira Anna Carbone and colleagues seeks to bridge this knowledge gap by investigating the efficacy and tolerability of naltrexone/bupropion (NB) extended release in treating pathological eating behaviors and promoting weight loss among obese patients with BED.

In this preliminary study, Carbone et al. recruited treatment-seeking obese individuals with and without BED from an Eating Disorder unit. The participants underwent comprehensive evaluations including psychiatric interviews, self-administered questionnaires assessing eating behaviors and mood disorders, and medical/nutritional assessments. Following these evaluations, patients began treatment with NB alongside prescribed lifestyle modifications. The study's design allowed for a thorough analysis of the effects of NB on weight loss and pathological eating behaviors over a 16-week period.

The main advances highlighted by Carbone et al.'s research include significant weight loss in both BED and non-BED groups, with improvements in pathological eating behaviors such as binge eating and emotional eating among BED patients. The study also notes the tolerability of NB, with side effects being manageable and not leading to treatment discontinuation in most cases. Looking forward, the authors suggest that future research should focus on long-term safety, efficacy of NB in maintaining weight loss, and its impact on BED-related medical complications. This preliminary evidence positions NB as a promising therapeutic option for obese BED patients resistant to traditional weight-loss programs.

Psychiatric Adverse Events and Effects on Mood with Prolonged-Release Naltrexone/Bupropion Combination Therapy: A Pooled Analysis [82]

This is a machine-generated summary of:

Pi-Sunyer, Xavier; Apovian, Caroline M.; McElroy, Susan L.; Dunayevich, Eduardo; Acevedo, Lisette M.; Greenway, Frank L.: Psychiatric adverse events and effects on mood with prolonged-release naltrexone/bupropion combination therapy: a pooled analysis [82]

Published in: International Journal of Obesity (2019)
Link to original: https://doi.org/10.1038/s41366-018-0302-z

If you want to cite the papers, please refer to the original.

For technical reasons we could not place the page where the original quote is coming from.

Research highlights

Introduction:

Excess body weight is a well-established risk factor for numerous health conditions, with even modest weight loss yielding significant health benefits. However, the psychiatric safety of weight management medications remains a concern, particularly given historical issues with centrally acting anti-obesity treatments. Now a new study by Xavier Pi-Sunyer and colleagues addresses these concerns by evaluating the psychiatric adverse effects (PAEs) associated with naltrexone/bupropion (NB), a medication approved for chronic weight management.

Main Body:

The research conducted by Pi-Sunyer et al. is a post hoc analysis of data pooled from placebo-controlled clinical trials, focusing on the psychiatric safety profile of NB. The study encompassed subjects with overweight or obesity, examining PAEs through various measures including the Inventory of Depressive Symptomatology Self-Report (IDS-SR) and the Columbia Classification Algorithm of Suicide Assessment (C-CASA). The methodology was robust, involving double-blind randomized trials with dose escalation and comprehensive criteria to minimize mood changes among participants.

Pi-Sunyer's team found that while PAEs occurred more frequently with NB compared to placebo, they were generally mild or moderate in severity and transient. Notably, the incidence of depression-related PAEs was lower in the NB group, and there was no association with increased suicidal ideation.

Conclusion:

The study by Pi-Sunyer et al. represents a significant advance in understanding the psychiatric safety of anti-obesity medications. It provides reassurance that NB does not significantly increase the risk of depression or suicidal thoughts compared to placebo. Looking forward, it is essential to continue monitoring patients for psychiatric symptoms and to further investigate NB's effects on individuals with existing depression or those on antidepressant medications.

Extended-Release Naltrexone/Bupropion Is Safe and Effective Among Subjects with Type 2 Diabetes Already Taking Incretin Agents: A Post-hoc Analysis of the LIGHT trial [83]

This is a machine-generated summary of:

Wharton, Sean; Yin, Peter; Burrows, Melonie; Gould, Errol; Blavignac, Jessica; Christensen, Rebecca A. G.; Kamran, Elham; Camacho, Fernando; Barakat, Maxime: Extended-release naltrexone/bupropion is safe and effective among subjects with type 2 diabetes already taking incretin agents: a post-hoc analysis of the LIGHT trial [83]

Published in: International Journal of Obesity (2021)

Link to original: https://doi.org/10.1038/s41366-021-00831-4

If you want to cite the papers, please refer to the original.

For technical reasons we could not place the page where the original quote is coming from.

Research highlights

Introduction:

Obesity significantly compounds the health challenges faced by individuals with type 2 diabetes, with a majority of this population grappling with overweight or obesity issues. Current clinical guidelines underscore the importance of weight management as a cornerstone for optimal glycemic control in diabetes care. Now a new study by Sean Wharton and colleagues delves into the effectiveness and safety of the combination medication extended-release naltrexone and bupropion (NB) for weight management in patients with type 2 diabetes who are concurrently on incretin-based therapies.

Main Body:

Wharton et al.'s research, a post-hoc analysis of the LIGHT trial, specifically targets the gap in knowledge regarding the concomitant use of NB with incretin agents such as dipeptidyl peptidase-4 inhibitors (DPP-4) or glucagon-like peptide-1 receptor agonists (GLP-1 RAs). The study meticulously sifts through data from subjects who were on either DPP-4 inhibitors or GLP-1 RAs at baseline, providing insights into weight change dynamics over time. The methodology employed mixed models to analyze weight changes or percentage change over time. Participants also engaged in a comprehensive web-based weight management program, reinforcing lifestyle interventions alongside medication.

Conclusion:

The study presents compelling evidence that NB is not only effective but also generally well-tolerated for inducing weight loss among patients with type 2 diabetes on incretin therapies. It highlights that NB's efficacy is maintained irrespective of concurrent incretin agent use, addressing a critical knowledge gap in diabetes and obesity treatment paradigms. This analysis paves the way for integrating NB into multifaceted treatment approaches for patients already receiving incretin-based glycemic management. Looking ahead, further research could explore NB's potential synergies with SGLT-2 inhibitors, another class of antihyperglycemic agents. In summary, Wharton and colleagues' work substantiates the role of NB as part of an evidence-based strategy for managing obesity in patients with type 2 diabetes on incretin therapies, marking a significant stride in holistic diabetic care.

Bibliography

1. Richard D, Picard F, Lemieux C, Lalonde J, Samson P, Deshaies Y. The effects of topiramate and sex hormones on energy balance of male and female rats. Int J Obes Relat Metab Disord. 2002;26:344–53.
2. Richard D, Ferland J, Lalonde J, Samson P, Deshaies Y. Influence of topiramate in the regulation of energy balance. Nutrition. 2000;16:961–6.
3. Arvaniti K, Richard D, Tremblay A. Reproducibility of energy and macronutrient intake and related substrate oxidation rates in a buffet-type meal. Br J Nutr. 2000;83:489–95.
4. Tremblay A, Poehlman ET, Després JP, Thériault G, Danforth E, Bouchard C. Endurance training with constant energy intake in identical twins: changes over time in energy expenditure and related hormones. Metabolism. 1997;46:499–503.
5. VIVUS. VIVUS Reports Topline Findings From FORTRESS. www.vivus.com, 21 Dec 2011. Media Release.
6. VIVUS Inc. VIVUS provides update on timing of European decision for Qnexa(R). www.vivus.com, 05 Jun 2012. Media Release.
7. VIVUS Inc. VIVUS provides update on the review of the Qsiva marketing authorization application. www.vivus.com, 21 Sep 2012. Media Release.
8. VIVUS Inc. VIVUS Announces Issuance of Key Patent for Qnexa(TM)—A Novel Therapy to Treat Obesity. www.vivus.com, 13 Jun 2006 Media Release.
9. Qsymia (phentermine and topiramate extended-release) capsules for oral use. US Prescribing Information. 2012.
10. Garvey WT, Troupin B, Day WW. Decreased progression to diabetes in subjects with prediabetes after 2 years of treatment with controlled-release phentermine/topiramate. 47th Annual Meeting of the European Association for the Study of Diabetes.: abstr. 907, 12 Sep 2011.
11. Garvey WT, Ryan DH, Look M, Gadde KM, Allison DB, Peterson CA, Schwiers M, Day WW, Bowden CH. Two-year sustained weight loss and metabolic benefits with controlled-release phentermine/topiramate in obese and overweight adults (SEQUEL): a randomized,

placebo-con-trolled, phase 3 extension study. Am J Clin Nutr. 2012;95:297–308. https://doi.org/10.3945/ajcn.111.024927.
12. Van Gaal LF, Cheskin LJ, Najarian T, et al. Long-term glycaemic effects of weight loss with low-dose, controlled-release phentermine/topiramate (PHEN/TPM CR) in overweight/obese subjects with diabetes. 47th Annual Meeting of the European Association for the Study of Diabetes.: abstr. 906, 12 Sep 2011.
13. Vivus. VIVUS and Alvogen announce marketing agreement for Qsymia® in the Republic of Korea [media release]. 5 Sep 2017. https://ir.vivus.com/news-releases/news-release-details/vivus-and-alvogen-announce-marketing-agreement-qsymiar-republic
14. Hsia DS, Gosselin NH, Williams J, et al. A randomized, double-blind, placebo-controlled, pharmacokinetic and pharmacodynamic study of a fixed-dose combination of phentermine/topiramate in adolescents with obesity. Diabetes Obes Metab. 2020;22(4):480–91.
15. VIVUS LLC. QSYMIA (phentermine and topiramate extended-release capsules): US prescribing information. 2022. https://www.accessdata.fda.gov/drugsatfda_docs/label/2022/022580s021lbl.pdf. Accessed 18 July 2022.
16. McCuen-Wurst C, Ruggieri M, Allison KC. Disordered eating and obesity: associations between binge-eating disorder, night-eating syndrome, and weight-related comorbidities. Ann N Y Acad Sci. 2018;1411(1):96–105.
17. Picot J, Jones J, Colquitt JL, Gospodarevskaya E, Loveman E, Baxter L et al. The clinical effectiveness and cost-effectiveness of bariatric (weight loss) surgery for obesity: a systematic review and economic evaluation. Health Technol Assess Winchester 2009; 13(41):1357 https://doi.org/10.3310/hta13410.
18. Padwal R, Li S, Lau D. Long-term pharmacotherapy for overweight and obesity: a systematic review and meta-analysis of randomized controlled trials. Int J Obes Relat Metab Disord. 2003;27:1437–46.
19. Padwal RS, Majumdar SR. Drug treatments for obesity: orlistat, sibutramine, and rimonabant. Lancet. 2007;369(9555):71–7.
20. Gadde KM, Allison DB, Ryan DH, Peterson CA, Troupin B, Schwiers ML, et al. Effects of low-dose, controlled-release, phentermine plus topiramate combination on weight and associated comorbidities in overweight and obese adults (CONQUER): a randomised, placebo-controlled, phase 3 trial. Lancet. 2011;377:1341–52.
21. Allison DB, Gadde KM, Garvey WT, Peterson CA, Schwiers ML, Najarian T, et al. Controlled-release phentermine/topiramate in severely obese adults: a randomized controlled trial (EQUIP). Obesity. 2012;20:330–42.
22. Fujioka K, Seaton TB, Rowe E, Jelinek CA, Raskin P, Lebovitz HE, et al. Weight loss with sibutramine improves glycaemic control and other metabolic parameters in obese patients with type 2 diabetes mellitus. Diabetes Obes Metab. 2000;2(3):175–87.
23. Aasprang A, Andersen JR, Vage V, Kolotkin RL, Natvig GK. Five-year changes in health-related quality of life after biliopancreatic diversion with duodenal switch. Obes Surg. 2013;23(10):1662–8.
24. Warkentin LM, Das D, Majumdar SR, Johnson JA, Padwal RS. The effect of weight loss on health-related quality of life: systematic review and meta-analysis of randomized trials. Obes Rev. 2014;15(3):169–82.
25. Maciejewski ML, Patrick DL, Williamson DF. A structured review of randomized controlled trials of weight loss showed little improvement in health-related quality of life. J Clin Epidemiol. 2005;58(6):568–78.
26. Kolotkin RL, Crosby RD, Kosloski KD, Williams GR. Development of a brief measure to assess quality of life in obesity. Obes Res. 2001;9(2):102–11.
27. Ware JE, Snow KK, Kosinski M, Gandek B. SF-36 health survey: manual and interpretation guide. Boston: Health Institute, New England Medical Center; 1993.
28. Kolotkin RL, Crosby RD. Psychometric evaluation of the impact of weight on quality of life-lite questionnaire (IWQOL-lite) in a community sample. Qual Life Res. 2002;11(2):157–71.

29. Hayes AF. Introduction to mediation, moderation, and conditional process analysis: a regression-based approach. NY: Guilford Press; 2013.
30. Padula WV, Allen RR, Nair KV. Determining the cost of obesity and its common comorbidities from a commercial claims database. Clin Obes. 2014;4:53–8.
31. Andreyeva T, Sturm R, Ringel JS. Moderate and severe obesity have large differences in health care costs. Obes Res. 2004;12(12):1936–43.
32. Quesenberry CP Jr, Caan B, Jacobson A. Obesity, health services use, and health care costs among members of a health maintenance organization. Arch Intern Med. 1998;158(5):466–72.
33. Neovius M, Narbro K. Cost-effectiveness of pharmacological anti-obesity treatments: a systematic review. Int J Obes. 2008;32(12):1752–63.
34. Woloshin S, Schwartz LM. The new weight-loss drugs, lorcaserin and phentermine-topiramate: slim pickings? JAMA Intern Med. 2014;174(4):615–9.
35. Jensen MD, Ryan DH, Apovian CM, Ard JD, Comuzzie AG, Donato KA, et al. AHA/ACC/TOS guideline for the management of overweight and obesity in adults: a report of the American College of Cardiology/American Heart Association Task Force on Practice Guidelines and the Obesity Society. J Am Coll Cardiol. 2014. 2013;63(25 Pt B):2985–3023.
36. Apovian CM, Aronne LJ, Bessesen DH, McDonnell ME, Murad MH, Pagotto U, et al. Pharmacological management of obesity: an endocrine society clinical practice guideline. J Clin Endocrinol Metab. 2015;100:342–62.
37. Contrave®. (naltrexone HCl and bupropion HCl) extended-release tablets: US prescribing information. Deerfield (IL): Takeda Pharmaceuticals America Inc.; 2014.
38. Mysimba. (naltrexone hydrochloride/bupropion hydrochloride) 8 mg/90 mg prolonged-release tablets: summary of product characteristics. London: European Medicines Agency; 2015.
39. Billes SK, Sinnayah P, Cowley MA. Naltrexone/bupropion for obesity: an investigational combination pharmacotherapy for weight loss. Pharmacol Res. 2014;84:1–11.
40. Greenway FL, Fujioka K, Plodkowski RA, Mudaliar S, Guttadauria M, Erickson J, et al. Effect of naltrexone plus bupropion on weight loss in overweight and obese adults (COR-I): a multicentre, randomised, double-blind, placebo-controlled, phase 3 trial. Lancet. 2010;376:595–605.
41. Wadden TA, Foreyt JP, Foster GD, Hill JO, Klein S, O'Neil PM, et al. Weight loss with naltrexone SR/bupropion SR combination therapy as an adjunct to behavior modification: the COR-BMOD trial. Obesity (Silver Spring). 2011;19(1):110–20.
42. Hollander P, Gupta AK, Plodkowski R, Greenway F, Bays H, Burns C, et al. Effects of naltrexone sustained-release/bupropion sustained-release combination therapy on body weight and glycemic parameters in overweight and obese patients with type 2 diabetes. Diabetes Care. 2013;36(12):4022–9.
43. Apovian CM, Aronne L, Rubino D, Still C, Wyatt H, Burns C, et al. A randomized, phase 3 trial of naltrexone SR/bupropion SR on weight and obesity-related risk factors (COR-II). Obesity (Silver Spring). 2013;21(5):935–43.
44. Plutzky J, Chilton R, Still C, et al. Weight loss, blood pressure, pulse and circadian patterns with naltrexone sustained-release/bupropion sustained-release combination therapy for obesity [abstract no. 1013–286]. J Am Coll Cardiol. 2011;57(14 Suppl):E517.
45. Takeda Pharmaceuticals America Inc. Contrave® (naltrexone HCl and bupropion HCl) extended-release tablets: US prescribing information. 2014. http://www.fda.gov. Accessed 8 June 2015.
46. Orexigen Therapeutics Ireland Ltd. Mysimba™ 8 mg/90 mg prolonged-release tablets: EU summary of product characteristics. 2015. http://www.ema.europe.eu. Accessed 8 June 2015.
47. World Health Organization. Obesity and overweight: fact sheet no. 311. 2015. http://www.who.int/mediacentre/factsheets. Accessed 8 June 2015.
48. National Institute for Health and Care Excellence. Obesity: identification, assessment and management of overweight and obesity in children, young people and adults. NICE clinical guideline 189. 2014. http://www.nice.org.uk/guidance. Accessed 8 June 2015.

49. Kolotkin RL, Burns C, Walsh B, et al. Combination naltrexone/bupropion therapy resulted in clinically meaningful improvements in weight and quality of life (QoL): integrated analysis of four phase 3 trials [abstract no. 1056-P]. Diabetes. 2013;62(Suppl 1):A272.
50. Cunningham JW, Wiviott SD. Modern obesity pharmacotherapy: weighing cardiovascular risk and benefit. Clin Cardiol. 2014;37(11):693–9.
51. Morton GJ, Meek TH, Schwartz MW. Neurobiology of food intake in health and disease. Nat Rev Neurosci. 2014;15:367–78. https://doi.org/10.1038/nrn3745.
52. Morton GJ, Blevins JE, Williams DL, et al. Leptin action in the forebrain regulates the hindbrain response to satiety signals. J Clin Invest. 2005;115:703–10. https://doi.org/10.1172/JCI22081.
53. Volkow ND, Wang G-J, Baler RD. Reward, dopamine and the control of food intake: implications for obesity. Trends Cogn Sci. 2011;15:37–46. https://doi.org/10.1016/j.tics.2010.11.001.
54. Caroleo M, Primerano A, Rania M, et al. A real world study on the genetic, cognitive and psychopathological differences of obese patients clustered according to eating behaviours. Eur Psychiatry. 2018;48:58–64. https://doi.org/10.1016/j.eurpsy.2017.11.009.
55. Greenway FL, Dunayevich E, Tollefson G, et al. Comparison of combined bupropion and naltrexone therapy for obesity with monotherapy and placebo. J Clin Endocrinol Metab. 2009;94(12):4898–906.
56. Smith SR, Fujioka K, Gupta AK, et al. Combination therapy with naltrexone and bupropion for obesity reduces total and visceral adiposity. Diabetes Obes Metab. 2013;15(9):863–6.
57. Sherman MM, Ungureanu S, Rey JA. Naltrexone/bupropion ER (Contrave): newly approved treatment option for chronic weight management in obese adults. P T. 2016;41:164–72.
58. Appolinario JC, Godoy-Matos A, Fontenelle LF, et al. An open-label trial of sibutramine in obese patients with binge-eating disorder. J Clin Psychiatry. 2002;63:28–30. https://doi.org/10.4088/JCP.v63n0106.
59. Pataky Z, Gasteyger C, Ziegler O, et al. Efficacy of rimonabant in obese patients with binge eating disorder. Exp Clin Endocrinol Diabetes. 2013;121:20–6. https://doi.org/10.1055/s-0032-1329957.
60. Smith SR, Blundell JE, Burns C, et al. Pramlintide treatment reduces 24-h caloric intake and meal sizes and improves control of eating in obese subjects: a 6-wk translational research study. Am J Physiol Endocrinol Metab. 2007;293:E620–7. https://doi.org/10.1152/ajpendo.00217.2007.
61. Yanovski SZ, Yanovski JA. Naltrexone-extended release plus bupropion-extended release for treatment of obesity. JAMA. 2015;313:1213–4.
62. Ali KF, Shukla AP, Aronne LJ. Bupropion-SR plus naltrexone-SR for the treatment of mild-to-moderate obesity. Expert Rev Clin Pharmacol. 2016;9:27–34. https://doi.org/10.1586/17512433.2016.1100072.
63. Ryan DH, Yockey SR. Weight loss and improvement in comorbidity: differences at 5, 10, 15%, and over. Curr Obes Rep. 2017;6:187–94.
64. Wing RR, Lang W, Wadden TA, Safford M, Knowler WC, Bertoni AG, et al. Benefits of modest weight loss in improving cardiovascular risk factors in overweight and obese individuals with type 2 diabetes. Diabetes Care. 2011;34(7):1481–6.
65. Astrup A, Greenway FL, Ling W, Pedicone L, Lachowicz J, Strader CD, et al. Randomized controlled trials of the D1/D5 antagonist ecopipam for weight loss in obese subjects. Obesity. 2007;15:1717–31.
66. Luppino FS, de Wit LM, Bouvy PF, Stijnen T, Cuijpers P, Penninx BW, et al. Overweight, obesity, and depression: a systematic review and meta-analysis of longitudinal studies. Arch Gen Psychiatry. 2010;67:220–9.
67. Reeves RR, Ladner ME. Antidepressant-induced suicidality: an update. CNS Neurosci Ther. 2010;16:227–34.
68. Wightman DS, Foster VJ, Krishen A, Richard NE. Modell JG meta-analysis of suicidality in placebo-controlled clinical trials of adults taking bupropion. Prime care companion. J Clin Psychiatry. 2010;12:12.e1–8.

69. McElroy SL, Guerdjikova AI, Kim DD, Burns C, Harris-Collazo R, Landbloom R, et al. Naltrexone/bupropion combination therapy in overweight or obese patients with major depressive disorder: results of a pilot study. Prime Care Companion CNS Disord. 2013;15
70. Nissen SE, Wolski KE, Prcela L, Wadden TA, Buse JB, Bakris G, et al. Effect of naltrexone-bupropion on major adverse cardiovascular events in overweight and obese patients with cardiovascular risk factors: a randomized clinical trial. JAMA. 2016;315:990–1004.
71. Boehringer Ingelheim Pharmaceuticals, Inc. JARDIANCE® (empagliflozin) prescribing information (revised). 2020.
72. Tremblay A, Chaput J-P, Bérubé-Parent S, Prud'homme D, Leblanc C, Alméras N, Després J-P. The effect of topiramate on energy balance in obese men: a 6-month double-blind randomized placebo-controlled study with a 6-month open-label extension. Eur J Clin Pharmacol. 2007;63:123–34. https://doi.org/10.1007/s00228-006-0220-1.
73. Cameron F, Whiteside G, McKeage K. Phentermine and Topiramate extended release (Qsymia™). Drugs. 2012;72:2033–42. https://doi.org/10.2165/11640860-000000000-00000.
74. Dhillo S. Phentermine/Topiramate: pediatric first approval. Pediatr Drugs. 2022;24:715–20. https://doi.org/10.1007/s40272-022-00532-z.
75. Grunvald E, DeConde J. Phentermine–topiramate extended release for the dual treatment of obesity and sleep-related eating disorder: a case report. J Med Case Rep. 2022;16:34. https://doi.org/10.1186/s13256-021-03250-1.
76. Finkelstein EA, Kruger E, Karnawat S. Cost-effectiveness analysis of Qsymia for weight loss. Pharmaco Economics. 2014;33:699–706. https://doi.org/10.1007/s40273-014-0182-6.
77. Kolotkin RL, Gadde KM, Peterson CA, Crosby RD. Health-related quality of life in two randomized controlled trials of phentermine/topiramate for obesity: what mediates improvement? Qual Life Res. 2015;25:1237–44. https://doi.org/10.1007/s11136-015-1153-x.
78. Li J, Reaven NL, Funk SE, McGaughey K, Neovius M. 4-year cost trajectories in real-world patients matched to the metabolic profiles of trial subjects before/after treatment with phentermine-topiramate. Drugs—Real World Outcomes. 2015;2:143–51. https://doi.org/10.1007/s40801-015-0021-x.
79. Greig SL, Keating GM. Naltrexone ER/bupropion ER in obesity management: a guide to its use. Drug Therap Perspect. 2015;31:417–24. https://doi.org/10.1007/s40267-015-0253-6.
80. Greig SL, Keating GM. Naltrexone ER/bupropion ER: a review in obesity management. Drugs. 2015;75:1269–80. https://doi.org/10.1007/s40265-015-0427-5.
81. Carbone EA, Caroleo M, Rania M, Calabrò G, Staltari FA, de Filippis R, Aloi M, Condoleo F, Arturi F, Segura-Garcia C. An open-label trial on the efficacy and tolerability of naltrexone/bupropion SR for treating altered eating behaviours and weight loss in binge eating disorder. Eat Weight Disord. 2020;26:779–88. https://doi.org/10.1007/s40519-020-00910-x.
82. Pi-Sunyer X, Apovian CM, McElroy SL, Dunayevich E, Acevedo LM, Greenway FL. Psychiatric adverse events and effects on mood with prolonged-release naltrexone/bupropion combination therapy: a pooled analysis. Int J Obes. 2019;43:2085–94. https://doi.org/10.1038/s41366-018-0302-z.
83. Wharton S, Yin P, Burrows M, Gould E, Blavignac J, Christensen RAG, Kamran E, Camacho F, Barakat M. Extended-release naltrexone/bupropion is safe and effective among subjects with type 2 diabetes already taking incretin agents: a post-hoc analysis of the LIGHT trial. Int J Obes. 2021;45:1687–95. https://doi.org/10.1038/s41366-021-00831-4.

Chapter 4
Role of Incretin Mimetics in the Management of Obesity

Shilpa Chugh Garcha and Sanjay Kalra

Gut hormones are known to play a critical role in the regulation of appetite and energy expenditure. Some of the important hormones that have been explored in the management of obesity includes ghrelin, glucagon-like peptide 1 (GLP-1), peptide tyrosine-tyrosine, oxyntomodulin, glicentin, pancreatic polypeptide, amylin, and cholecystokinin. Imbalance in the level of these hormones likely contributes to the development of obesity. The role of these gut hormones has received a lot of attention in the last few years as important therapeutic targets in the management of obesity.

In this chapter, the first study included explores the role of several hormones that are released from the gut in response to food and influence food intake and energy expenditure and underscores their importance in maintaining energy homeostasis. It also explores how the levels of these hormones are dysregulated in obesity.

Incretins are natural gut derived peptide hormones and mainly includes two incretins: glucagon-like peptide 1 (GLP-1) and glucose-dependent insulinotropic peptide (GIP) and medications that act through these incretin hormones are known as incretin-based therapies. GLP-1 is one of the most important gut hormones released in response to food intake and has been studied widely.

Glucagon-like peptide-1 receptor agonists commonly known as GLP-1 agonists are a class of drugs that have been successfully used in the treatment of type 2 diabetes. Now, three GLP-1 agonists liraglutide, semaglutide, and tirzepatide have received USFDA approval for use in patients who are overweight and obese. These are being extensively studied for their role in management of individuals who are overweight and obese and for their effect on cardiometabolic risk factors and other comorbidities such as sleep apnea.

S. C. Garcha (✉)
Sonepat, Haryana, India

S. Kalra
Department of Endocrinology, Bharti Hospital, Karnal, Haryana, India

S. C. Garcha, S. Kalra (eds.), *Drugs for Medical Management of Obesity*,
https://doi.org/10.1007/978-981-96-1651-0_4

Liraglutide 3.0 mg as a subcutaneous injection is approved by FDA as an adjunct to reduced-calorie diet and increased physical activity for chronic weight management in adults with an initial body mass index (BMI) of ≥30 kg/m^2 (obese) or ≥27 kg/m^2 (overweight) in the presence of at least one weight-related comorbidity. It has also been approved recently for pediatric patients ≥12 years and body weight >60 kg and an initial BMI corresponding to 30 kg/m^2 for adults (obese) by international cut-offs [1].

In this chapter, two studies have been included on the role of liraglutide in the management of overweight and obesity. One of the studies explores the efficacy and safety of liraglutide in obese and overweight individuals as seen in various clinical trials and the impact of liraglutide on biomarkers of cardiovascular risk. This study also highlighted the effect of weight loss by liraglutide on sleep apnea in obese individuals. Another study explored the effects of liraglutide along with behavioural therapy on hunger, fullness, cravings, and food preoccupation and its effects on weight management.

Semaglutide is another GLP-1 receptor agonist approved by FDA for weight management for subcutaneous use as an adjunct to a reduced calorie diet and increased physical activity in adult patients with an initial BMI of ≥30 kg/m^2 (obesity) or ≥27 kg/m^2 (overweight) and at least one weight-related comorbidity and in pediatric patients of age ≥12 years with an initial BMI at the 95th percentile or more for age and sex [2].

One of the studies included is a meta-analysis of the clinical trials exploring the efficacy and safety of Semaglutide 2.4 mg including its effect on body weight, BMI, waist circumference, glycemic control, and blood pressure. Another study included is the STEP-5 trial which was a phase 3 randomised controlled trial that explored the change in weight with the use of semaglutide and its impact on cardiometabolic risk factors including waist circumference, lipid and HbA1c levels, and blood pressure.

One more study included here explores the role of Semaglutide in individuals with obesity phenotype of heart failure with preserved ejection fraction (HFpEF) without diabetes in STEP-HFpEF trial. The study also explores improvements in clinical outcomes which are associated with the degree of weight loss.

Recently, FDA has approved a dual GIP and GLP-1 receptor agonist tirzepatide, for the management of overweight and obesity. Tirzepatide was previously approved for the management of type 2 diabetes and now it is approved as an adjunct to a reduced-calorie diet and increased physical activity for chronic weight management in adults with an initial BMI of ≥30 kg/m2 (obesity) or ≥27 kg/m^2 (overweight) in the presence of at least one weight-related comorbid condition [3].

Meta-analysis of randomized controlled trials of tirzepatide shows that it significantly reduced body weight compared to placebo across various doses.

Incretin-mimetics have shown to play an important role in the management of obesity; however, they have been associated with various adverse events. One of the studies explored the adverse effects and gastrointestinal effects seen with this class of drugs such as nausea, vomiting, diarrhea, and constipation, which are most common and are key reason for discontinuation of the therapy. The study also addresses issues related to acute pancreatitis, and hepatic adverse events.

One of the studies included explores the effectiveness of these medications in individuals struggling to maintain their weight after bariatric surgery and supported the use of GLP-1 agonists in these individuals and they have shown efficacy and were associated with mild and transient gastrointestinal adverse effects.

Further research is going on to explore the use of these medications alone or in combination with other medications for the management of overweight and obesity and other related co-morbidities such as sleep apnea syndrome, non-alcoholic steatohepatitis, and cardiovascular health.

References for Introduction

(1) SAXENDA (liraglutide) injection, U.S. Food and Drug Administration website. https://www.accessdata.fda.gov/drugsatfda_docs/label/2023/206321s016lbl.pdf Revised Apr 2023. Accessed 8 Aug 2024
(2) WEGOVY (semaglutide) injection. U.S. Food and Drug Administration website. https://www.accessdata.fda.gov/drugsatfda_docs/label/2023/215256s007lbl.pdf Revised Jul 2023. Accessed 8 Aug 2024
(3) ZEPBOUND (tirzepatide) Injection. U.S. Food and Drug Administration website. https://www.accessdata.fda.gov/drugsatfda_docs/label/2024/217806s003lbl.pdf Revised Mar 2024. Accessed 8 Aug 2024.

4.1 Machine Generated Summaries

Disclaimer: The summaries in this chapter were generated from Springer Nature publications using abstractive AI auto-summarization: An abstraction-based summarizer creates new text based on deep learning. New phrases are created to summarize the content. As the constituted sentences are machine selected, they may not fully reflect the body of the work, so we strongly advise that the original content is read and cited. The auto-generated summaries were curated by the editor to meet Springer Nature publication standards.

Machine generated keywords: semaglutide, tirzepatide, liraglutide, glp, overweight obesity.

The Implication of Gut Hormones in the Regulation of Energy Homeostasis and Their Role in the Pathophysiology of Obesity [128]

This is a machine-generated summary of:

Koliaki, Chrysi; Liatis, Stavros; Dalamaga, Maria; Kokkinos, Alexander: The Implication of Gut Hormones in the Regulation of Energy Homeostasis and Their Role in the Pathophysiology of Obesity [128]

Published in: Current Obesity Reports (2020)

Link to original: https://doi.org/10.1007/s13679-020-00396-9

Copyright of the summarized publication:

If you want to cite the papers, please refer to the original.

For technical reasons we could not place the page where the original quote is coming from.

Research highlights

Background and Key Findings:

Obesity, a major health concern worldwide, is associated with numerous comorbidities that significantly impact life expectancy and healthcare systems. Characterized as a pandemic, its prevalence continues to rise despite extensive research and public health initiatives. A critical aspect of obesity is the regulation of energy homeostasis by neuronal networks that respond to various signals indicating energy availability. Now a new study by Chrysi Koliaki and colleagues delves into the intricate role of gut hormones in appetite regulation, energy balance, and their potential as therapeutic targets for obesity management.

Study Narrative:

Koliaki et al.'s comprehensive review examines how gut hormones, secreted in response to nutrient ingestion, influence eating behavior and energy homeostasis. These hormones include both orexigenic (ghrelin) and anorexigenic peptides (peptide tyrosine-tyrosine, GLP-1, oxyntomodulin, pancreatic polypeptide, amylin, cholecystokinin, Glicentin) that act on the central nervous system (CNS) to modulate food intake and energy expenditure.

The authors, acknowledges the challenges posed by their instability, which makes their plasma measurement difficult. They also explore the complex interactions between different gut hormones and how anorexigenic hormones can synergistically affect appetite suppression. Furthermore, the study investigates how obesity alters gut hormone profiles, leading to disrupted energy balance and perpetuating weight gain. The authors highlight adaptive changes in gut hormone levels following weight loss interventions like hypocaloric diets or bariatric surgery, noting distinct differences between these approaches.

Advances and Future Directions:

The main advances presented by Koliaki et al. include a detailed understanding of gut hormone interactions in regulating appetite and energy balance, as well as insights into how obesity can dysregulate these processes. The review points toward promising future directions in obesity treatment through gut hormone-based therapies that mimic post-bariatric surgery hormonal changes. According to the authors, combining multiple gut hormones could counteract the body's resistance to weight loss during dietary restriction. Such strategies could pave the way for "medical bypass" treatments as alternatives to surgery for a wider range of patients with obesity-related conditions. As Koliaki et al. suggest, further research is necessary to explore incretin physiology in individuals resistant to weight gain and the effects of gut hormones on thermogenesis, which could unlock new avenues for combating obesity.

Liraglutide: A Review of Its Use in the Management of Obesity [129]

This is a machine-generated summary of:

Scott, Lesley J.: Liraglutide: A Review of Its Use in the Management of Obesity [129]

Published in: Drugs (2015)

Link to original: https://doi.org/10.1007/s40265-015-0408-8

If you want to cite the papers, please refer to the original.

For technical reasons we could not place the page where the original quote is coming from.

Research highlights

Obesity has become a global health crisis, with the prevalence of overweight and obese individuals more than doubling since 1980. As of 2008, approximately 1.4 billion adults were overweight (defined by WHO as a body mass index (BMI) of ≥ 25 kg/m^2), and of these, around 500 million were obese (defined by WHO as a BMI of ≥ 30 kg/m^2). Obesity significantly increases the risk of various diseases, including diabetes, cardiovascular disorders, and certain cancers, and is associated with higher mortality rates for BMIs over the range of 22.5–25 kg/m^2.

Despite lifestyle interventions such as diet and exercise being fundamental to obesity management, many individuals require additional pharmacological or surgical interventions to achieve meaningful weight loss. Now a new study by Lesley J. Scott delves into the efficacy and safety of liraglutide 3 mg dose, a pharmacological agent targeting the incretin hormone glucagon-like peptide-1 (GLP-1), for chronic bodyweight management in obese or overweight adults with weight-related comorbidities.

This study provides a comprehensive review of liraglutide's pharmacology, its impact on bodyweight management, and its tolerability profile. Liraglutide is an acylated GLP-1 analogue that mimics the action of endogenous GLP-1 by binding to GLP-1 receptors and activating them. This activation leads to several physiological responses that contribute to weight loss, such as decreased calorie intake and improved eating behavior without increasing 24-hour energy expenditure. The study methodically analyzed data from phase II and III clinical trials focusing on liraglutide's effects on bodyweight in non-diabetic obese adults as well as those with type 2 diabetes.

The main advances highlighted in this study include significant reductions in bodyweight and improvements in various cardiometabolic biomarkers associated with cardiovascular risk when using liraglutide compared to placebo.

Additionally, liraglutide showed benefits in managing obstructive sleep apnoea severity due to weight loss in non-diabetic obese adults.

Looking forward, Scott et al. suggest that while the current data are promising for liraglutide as an effective weight management tool, further research is needed to fully understand its long-term impact on cardiovascular morbidity and mortality.

The authors also emphasize the importance of monitoring for potential adverse effects such as pancreatitis and thyroid cancer during treatment.

Effects of Liraglutide on Appetite, Food Preoccupation, and Food Liking: Results of a Randomized Controlled Trial [130]

This is a machine-generated summary of:

Tronieri, Jena Shaw; Wadden, Thomas A.; Walsh, Olivia; Berkowitz, Robert I.; Alamuddin, Naji; Gruber, Kathryn; Leonard, Sharon; Bakizada, Zayna M.; Chao, Ariana M.: Effects of liraglutide on appetite, food preoccupation, and food liking: results of a randomized controlled trial [130]

Published in: International Journal of Obesity (2019)

Link to original: https://doi.org/10.1038/s41366-019-0348-6

If you want to cite the papers, please refer to the original.

For technical reasons we could not place the page where the original quote is coming from.

Research highlights

Introduction:

Obesity remains a significant public health challenge, with behavioral treatment and pharmacotherapy each offering partial solutions. While behavioral interventions focus on modifying the external food environment, centrally acting pharmacological agents act on the internal environment to suppress appetite. Now a new study by Jena Shaw Tronieri and colleagues delves into the combined effects of intensive behavioral therapy (IBT) and liraglutide, a GLP-1 receptor agonist, on appetite control over a prolonged period.

Main Body:

Tronieri's team conducted a 52-week randomized controlled trial to assess changes in hunger, fullness, food preoccupation, cravings, and meal enjoyment among obese patients undergoing different treatment modalities. Participants received either IBT alone, IBT with liraglutide injections, or a multi-component approach that included a portion-controlled diet. The study's robust design involved regular appetite assessments using visual analogue scales and body weight measurements to track progress. The authors hypothesized that the combination of IBT and liraglutide would lead to greater improvements in appetite control. Indeed, initial findings supported this, with the IBT-liraglutide group reporting more significant reductions in hunger and increases in post-meal fullness than those receiving IBT alone.

Conclusion:

The study's main advance lies in demonstrating that adding liraglutide to behavioral therapy compared to behavioral therapy alone causes initial improvements in hunger, post meal fullness, and food preoccupation and suggests that it enhances early weight loss by improving appetite control. However, these benefits seemed to wane over time, with no significant differences in appetite measures between groups at one year. As per the study, while liraglutide's impact on appetite may diminish, its weight control effects persist. Future research should explore the long-term mechanisms of GLP-1 agonists' by which it helps in weight maintenance despite apparent decrease of its effect on appetite.

Efficacy and Safety of Once-Weekly Semaglutide in Adults with Overweight or Obesity: A Meta-Analysis [131]

This is a machine-generated summary of:

Zhong, Ping; Zeng, Hai; Huang, Miaochun; Fu, Wenbin; Chen, Zhixia: Efficacy and safety of once-weekly semaglutide in adults with overweight or obesity: a meta-analysis [131]

Published in: Endocrine (2022)

Link to original: https://doi.org/10.1007/s12020-021-02945-1

If you want to cite the papers, please refer to the original.

For technical reasons we could not place the page where the original quote is coming from.

Research highlights

Introduction:

Obesity is a growing global public health challenge, with an estimated prevalence affecting millions and contributing to various non-communicable diseases. Despite the availability of interventions, the need for more effective treatments remains pressing. Now a new study by Ping Zhong and colleagues conducted the first meta-analysis to evaluate the efficacy and safety of once-weekly subcutaneous semaglutide in adults with overweight or obesity.

Main Body:

Zhong et al. meticulously followed the Preferred Reporting Items for Systematic Reviews and Meta-Analyses (PRISMA) guidelines to search databases like PubMed, Embase, and the Cochrane Library for randomized controlled trials (RCTs) comparing once-weekly semaglutide with placebo. The inclusion criteria were strict, focusing on adults with a body-mass index of 27 kg/m^2 or higher without diabetes, and studies had to last at least 20 weeks. The team extracted data on various outcomes ranging from weight change, cardiometabolic risk profiles to health-related quality of life measures.

The meta-analysis included four high-quality RCTs with low risk of bias, involving a total of 3447 patients. The results were clear: once-weekly semaglutide significantly outperformed placebo in reducing body weight, BMI, waist circumference, and improving glycemic control and blood pressure. The authors noted that the magnitude of weight loss observed was clinically meaningful and emphasized the potential of semaglutide as a promising therapy in managing obesity.

Conclusion:

The study by Zhong et al. marks a significant advance in obesity treatment, demonstrating that once-weekly semaglutide offers substantial benefits over placebo in weight management and associated health outcomes. The study supports the use of semaglutide 2.4 mg as an effective therapeutic option for adults struggling with obesity. Looking ahead, the authors suggest that future research should focus on long-term cardiovascular outcomes trials to further establish the cardiovascular benefits of semaglutide.

Two-Year Effects of Semaglutide in Adults with Overweight or Obesity: The STEP 5 Trial [132]

This is a machine-generated summary of:

Garvey, W. Timothy; Batterham, Rachel L.; Bhatta, Meena; Buscemi, Silvio; Christensen, Louise N.; Frias, Juan P.; Jódar, Esteban; Kandler, Kristian; Rigas, Georgia; Wadden, Thomas A.; Wharton, Sean: Two-year effects of semaglutide in adults with overweight or obesity: the STEP 5 trial [132]

Published in: Nature Medicine (2022)

Link to original: https://doi.org/10.1038/s41591-022-02026-4

If you want to cite the papers, please refer to the original.

For technical reasons we could not place the page where the original quote is coming from.

Research highlights

Background and Key Findings:

The global prevalence of overweight and obesity has escalated to epidemic proportions, with behavioral interventions such as diet and exercise modifications being the cornerstone of treatment. Despite these efforts, achieving long-term, clinically meaningful weight loss remains a challenge, leading to the incorporation of pharmacotherapy as an adjunct for individuals with a body mass index (BMI) $\geq$30 kg/m^2, or $\geq$27 kg/m^2 with comorbidities. Now a new study by W. Timothy Garvey and colleagues has extended the understanding of long-term weight management through pharmacological means by evaluating the efficacy of semaglutide—a glucagon-like peptide-1 analog—in conjunction with behavioral intervention over a two-year period.

Study Narrative:

The STEP 5 trial, a phase 3, randomized, double-blind, placebo-controlled multinational study, is the longest to date in assessing semaglutide's role in weight management. From October 2018 to February 2019, participants were assigned to receive either semaglutide 2.4 mg or placebo weekly. The trial's robust design included two estimands to assess efficacy: the 'treatment policy' estimand for all participants regardless of adherence or intervention changes and the 'trial product' estimand assuming perfect adherence. The primary endpoints were percentage change in body weight from baseline to week 104 and achievement of ≥5% weight loss at week 104.

Garvey et al.'s findings were significant: participants on semaglutide experienced an average weight reduction of 15.2%, markedly surpassing placebo results. Moreover, semaglutide users were more likely to achieve weight loss thresholds of 10%, 15%, and 20%. The study also noted improvements in cardiometabolic risk factors such as waist circumference, lipid levels, HbA1c levels, and blood pressure.

Advances and Future Directions:

The STEP 5 trial represents a major advance in obesity pharmacotherapy by demonstrating that semaglutide can induce substantial weight loss that is sustainable over two years when combined with lifestyle intervention. Our findings support the benefit of continued semaglutide treatment for sustained weight loss, the author remarks.

Looking ahead, the implications for improving obesity-related health outcomes are considerable. The study suggests that semaglutide may also positively impact glycemic status, however, to understand its role in delaying or preventing type 2 diabetes onset—further research is needed to confirm this benefit. As obesity continues to be a significant public health concern, Garvey's work underscores the importance of ongoing innovation in treatment strategies that offer hope for better disease management.

Semaglutide in HFpEF Across Obesity Class and by Body Weight Reduction: A Prespecified Analysis of the STEP-HFpEF Trial [133]

This is a machine-generated summary of:

Borlaug, Barry A.; Kitzman, Dalane W.; Davies, Melanie J.; Rasmussen, Søren; Barros, Eric; Butler, Javed; Einfeldt, Mette Nygaard; Hovingh, G. Kees; Møller, Daniél Vega; Petrie, Mark C.; Shah, Sanjiv J.; Verma, Subodh; Abhayaratna, Walter; Ahmed, Fozia Z.; Chopra, Vijay; Ezekowitz, Justin; Fu, Michael; Ito, Hiroshi; Lelonek, Małgorzata; Melenovsky, Vojtech; Núñez, Julio; Perna, Eduardo; Schou, Morten; Senni, Michele; van der Meer, Peter; Von Lewinski, Dirk; Wolf, Dennis; Kosiborod, Mikhail N.: Semaglutide in HFpEF across obesity class and by body weight reduction: a prespecified analysis of the STEP-HFpEF trial [133]

Published in: Nature Medicine (2023)

Link to original: https://doi.org/10.1038/s41591-023-02526-x

Copyright of the summarized publication:

If you want to cite the papers, please refer to the original.

For technical reasons we could not place the page where the original quote is coming from.

Research highlights

Research Highlight for Nature Journal

Background and Key Findings:

Heart failure with preserved ejection fraction (HFpEF) is a growing global health concern, particularly its obesity phenotype, which presents with more severe symptoms and higher hospitalization risks. Despite the increasing prevalence, treatment options remain limited. Now a new study by Barry A. Borlaug and colleagues addresses this challenge by examining the efficacy of semaglutide, a glucagon-like peptide-1 receptor agonist, in patients with HFpEF across varying classes of obesity.

Study Insights:

The STEP-HFpEF trial revealed that weekly treatment with 2.4 mg of semaglutide significantly improved symptoms, physical limitations, exercise function, and reduced inflammation while promoting weight loss compared to placebo. The study spanned from March 2021 to March 2022, enrolling patients who were then randomized to receive either semaglutide or placebo. Notably, the benefits of semaglutide were consistent across all obesity classes without heterogeneity in treatment effects. Furthermore, a greater degree of weight loss was associated with more pronounced improvements in clinical outcomes.

Borlaug's team employed rigorous methods to ensure robust results. Patients were stratified by obesity class and changes in body weight were meticulously recorded and analyzed. The study's comprehensive approach included both intention-to-treat and on-treatment analyses, revealing that larger reduction in body weight correlated with greater improvements in clinical measures such as the Kansas City Cardiomyopathy Questionnaire-Clinical Summary Score (KCCQ-CSS), change in 6-minute walk distance (6MWD) and C-reactive protein levels.

Advances and Future Directions:

This research marks a significant advance in treating HFpEF patients with obesity, demonstrating that semaglutide-induced weight loss is beneficial across all obesity categories. The findings underscore the importance of weight reduction as an effective intervention for this patient group. Semaglutide mediated weight loss is a key therapeutic strategy for patients with obesity phenotype of HfpEF as per the study.

Further trials are set to explore long-term effects and potential synergies with other treatments such as sodium-glucose co-transporter-2 inhibitors. While the study focused on non-diabetic patients, ongoing trials are set to evaluate semaglutide's impact on those with diabetes. Also, limited insights are available on how semaglutide influences visceral fat loss and its association with clinical improvements—a crucial aspect considering BMI's limitations as an adiposity measure.

In conclusion, Borlaug et al.'s work offers compelling evidence supporting semaglutide as a transformative treatment for HFpEF associated with obesity.

Efficacy and Safety of the Dual GIP and GLP-1 Receptor Agonist Tirzepatide for Weight Loss: A Meta-Analysis of Randomized Controlled Trials [134]

This is a machine-generated summary of:

de Mesquita, Yasmin Luz Lima; Pera Calvi, Izabela; Reis Marques, Isabela; Almeida Cruz, Sara; Padrao, Eduardo Messias Hirano; Carvalho, Pedro Emanuel de Paula; da Silva, Caroliny Hellen Azevedo; Cardoso, Rhanderson; Moura, Filipe Azevedo; Rafalskiy, Vladimir Vitalievich: Efficacy and safety of the dual GIP and GLP-1 receptor agonist tirzepatide for weight loss: a meta-analysis of randomized controlled trials [134]

Published in: International Journal of Obesity (2023)

Link to original: https://doi.org/10.1038/s41366-023-01337-x

If you want to cite the papers, please refer to the original.

For technical reasons we could not place the page where the original quote is coming from.

Research highlights

Introduction:

The global rise in obesity rates has become a pressing public health issue, with projections indicating that by 2030, a staggering number of women and men will be affected by obesity, totaling approximately 1,02 billion individuals worldwide. This condition is linked to an array of life-threatening diseases, including cardiovascular ailments, type 2 diabetes, and various cancers. Traditional non-invasive treatments have largely revolved around lifestyle changes, with limited long-term pharmacological options available. Now a new study by Yasmin Luz Lima Mesquita et al. has explored the efficacy of tirzepatide, a novel dual GIP and GLP-1 receptor agonist, in promoting weight loss among individuals with and without diabetes.

Main Body:

Mesquita and colleagues conducted a systematic review and meta-analysis of randomized controlled trials (RCTs) to assess the impact of tirzepatide on weight loss. Their rigorous methodology included stringent eligibility criteria for study inclusion and comprehensive searches across multiple databases. The team extracted data meticulously, resolving any discrepancies through consensus. They employed advanced statistical analyses to ensure robust results, accounting for potential biases and heterogeneity among the studies. The meta-analysis revealed that tirzepatide significantly reduced body weight compared to placebo across all doses tested.

Conclusion:

The research by Mesquita et al. marks a significant advance in obesity treatment options, demonstrating that tirzepatide can lead to considerable weight loss in patients with or without diabetes. While the drug was associated with increased gastrointestinal side effects, its benefits in weight management are clear. Long-term cardiovascular outcomes associated with tirzepatide use needs to be determined to fully understand its potential as a therapeutic agent in combating obesity-related health risks. As quoted by the authors, "The drug's risk-to-benefit with each dose should be evaluated in an individualized manner in clinical practice," underscoring the importance of personalized medicine in addressing this complex condition.

Efficacy and Safety of Tirzepatide for Treatment of Overweight or Obesity. A Systematic Review and Meta-Analysis [135]

This is a machine-generated summary of:

Tan, Bryan; Pan, Xin-Hui; Chew, Han Shi Jocelyn; Goh, Rachel Sze Jen; Lin, Chaoxing; Anand, Vickram Vijay; Lee, Ethan Cheng Zhe; Chan, Kai En; Kong, Gwyneth; Ong, Christen En Ya; Chung, Hui Charlotte; Young, Dan Yock; Chan, Mark Y.; Khoo, Chin Meng; Mehta, Anurag; Muthiah, Mark Dhinesh; Noureddin, Mazen; Ng, Cheng Han; Chew, Nicholas W. S.; Chin, Yip Han: Efficacy and safety of tirzepatide for treatment of overweight or obesity. A systematic review and meta-analysis [135]

Published in: International Journal of Obesity (2023)

Link to original: https://doi.org/10.1038/s41366-023-01321-5

If you want to cite the papers, please refer to the original.

For technical reasons we could not place the page where the original quote is coming from.

Research highlights

Introduction:

Obesity is a global health crisis, with a significant portion of the world's population grappling with overweight and obesity-related health issues. This multifaceted disease elevates the risk of numerous life-threatening conditions, including cardiometabolic diseases, type 2 diabetes mellitus, stroke, non-alcoholic fatty liver disease, and various cancers, leading to diminished quality of life for those affected. Despite existing treatments focusing on lifestyle changes, pharmacotherapy, and surgery, there remains a need for more effective interventions. Now a new study by Bryan Tan et al. has conducted a comprehensive systematic review and meta-analysis to evaluate the efficacy and safety of tirzepatide—a dual GIP/GLP-1 agonist—in individuals with obesity.

Methods:

Tan and colleagues meticulously searched databases such as Medline, Embase, and Cochrane CENTRAL for randomized controlled trials (RCTs) assessing tirzepatide's weight loss efficacy in obese patients. They employed rigorous inclusion criteria and extracted data on various outcomes including weight loss percentages, changes in BMI, waist circumference, lipid and glucose profiles, blood pressure, and adverse events. The team utilized advanced statistical tools in RStudio to perform meta-analyses. They also conducted sensitivity analyses to refine their findings further.

Results and Discussion:

The study's findings are groundbreaking; tirzepatide significantly outperformed placebos and the GLP-1 agonist semaglutide in promoting weight loss among participants. A dose-dependent relationship was evident with tirzepatide's efficacy in reducing body weight and improving metabolic parameters such as lipid profiles and glycemic control. These results suggest that tirzepatide could revolutionize the management of obesity by offering a more holistic approach to treating metabolic syndrome components simultaneously.

Tan et al.'s research indicates that tirzepatide may be superior to current FDA-approved obesity treatments due to its dual mechanism of action on incretin hormones. The study also points toward future research directions, including tirzepatide's potential impact on non-alcoholic fatty liver disease (NAFLD) and cardiovascular health. While acknowledging limitations such as potential adverse events—which were comparable to other treatments—the authors advocate for tirzepatide as a promising new therapy for obesity management.

In conclusion, this comprehensive analysis by Bryan Tan et al. provides compelling evidence for the effectiveness of tirzepatide in treating obesity. It opens avenues for future research into its broader metabolic impacts while positioning tirzepatide as an innovative treatment option for obesity.

What Is the Evidence Regarding the Safety of New Obesity Pharmacotherapies [136]

This is a machine-generated summary of:

Vidal, Josep; Flores, Lílliam; Jiménez, Amanda; Pané, Adriana; de Hollanda, Ana: What is the evidence regarding the safety of new obesity pharmacotherapies [136].

Published in: International Journal of Obesity (2024)
Link to original: https://doi.org/10.1038/s41366-024-01488-5

If you want to cite the papers, please refer to the original.

For technical reasons we could not place the page where the original quote is coming from.

Research highlights

Introduction:

The global obesity epidemic has led to a surge in the use of gut-hormone receptor agonists, such as GLP-1 receptor agonists, for weight management in people living with obesity (PLWO). These agents have shown promise in achieving significant weight loss when combined with lifestyle modifications. However, the long-term safety of these therapies remains a critical concern due to the chronic nature of obesity and the potential for extended drug exposure. Now, a new study by Josep Vidal and colleagues provides a comprehensive narrative review summarizing the safety evidence for gut-hormone receptor-based therapies, drawing primarily from phase 3 randomized clinical trials and the Semaglutide Effects on Cardiovascular Outcomes in People with Overweight or Obesity (SELECT) trial.

Main Body:

Vidal et al.'s review meticulously examines the safety profiles of liraglutide, semaglutide, and tirzepatide—key players in this drug class. The authors note that gastrointestinal adverse effects (AEs), such as nausea, vomiting, diarrhea, and constipation are the most commonly reported issues but are generally mild to moderate in severity. Importantly, they highlight that weight loss associated with these drugs is largely independent of gastrointestinal AEs. The review also addresses concerns about gallbladder-related AEs, acute pancreatitis, and hepatic Aes and various other health conditions, providing insights into their incidence rates and potential underlying mechanisms. The authors incorporate quotes from their findings to emphasize points such as the nuanced relationship between these therapies and acute pancreatitis: "The association between gut-hormone-based therapies and the occurrence of AP is a matter of controversy." Furthermore, they delve into strategies to mitigate AEs and discuss recent recommendations for patients undergoing procedures requiring anesthesia while on these medications.

Conclusion:

The main advance underscored by Vidal et al. is the affirmation of the safety profile of gut-hormone receptor agonists based on current evidence from clinical trials. They point out that while gastrointestinal AEs were a primary reason for discontinuation in some trials, overall data support the safe use of this drug family for treating obesity. They advocate for ongoing vigilance in monitoring AEs and call for future research to further clarify long-term safety implications. As the author puts it: "Further studies, and continuous surveillance are required to further refine the proper use of these new-obesity pharmacotherapies."

Efficacy of the Glucagon-like Peptide-1 Receptor Agonists Liraglutide and Semaglutide for the Treatment of Weight Regain After Bariatric Surgery: A Retrospective Observational Study [137]

This is a machine-generated summary of:

Jensen, Anders Boisen; Renström, Frida; Aczél, Stefan; Folie, Patrick; Biraima-Steinemann, Magdalena; Beuschlein, Felix; Bilz, Stefan: Efficacy of the Glucagon-Like Peptide-1 Receptor Agonists Liraglutide and Semaglutide for the Treatment of Weight Regain After Bariatric surgery: a Retrospective Observational Study [137]

Published in: Obesity Surgery (2023)

Link to original: https://doi.org/10.1007/s11695-023-06484-8

If you want to cite the papers, please refer to the original.

For technical reasons we could not place the page where the original quote is coming from.

Research highlights

Introduction:

Bariatric surgery stands as the most effective intervention for severe obesity, yet a significant proportion of patients experience substantial weight regain post-surgery, undermining its long-term benefits. Despite various interventions ranging from lifestyle modifications to pharmacotherapy, a definitive standard treatment for post-bariatric weight regain remains elusive. Now a new study by Anders Boisen Jensen and colleagues sheds light on the potential of glucagon-like peptide-1 receptor agonists (GLP-1 RAs) in addressing this challenge, presenting evidence from a retrospective observational study on the efficacy of liraglutide and semaglutide in a real-world patient setting.

Main Body:

Jensen et al. embarked on a meticulous journey to explore the effectiveness of GLP-1 RAs in patients grappling with weight regain after bariatric surgery. The study, conducted at the Cantonal Hospital of St. Gallen, Switzerland, retrospectively analyzed medical records of patients who had been prescribed GLP-1 RA therapy. The researchers meticulously collected data on changes in body weight and BMI over six months with GLP-1 therapy, alongside any adverse events related to the treatment. The aim of the study was to document the real-world efficacy and safety of prescribing both liraglutide and semaglutide for this patient group. The study's robust design included sensitivity analyses to account for factors such as time since surgery, type of GLP-1 RA used, and patient demographics and various other factors.

Conclusion:

The findings from Jensen's team are promising, indicating that both liraglutide and semaglutide can lead to significant weight loss in patients experiencing weight regain after bariatric surgery. The author notes that more than three-quarters of the patients lost over 5% of their baseline body weight. Underscoring the potential impact of GLP-1 RAs in clinical practice. While adverse events were reported, they were predominantly mild and transient gastrointestinal issues. Looking ahead, the authors call for randomized clinical trials to confirm these results and support the use of GLP-1 RAs as a treatment option for post-bariatric weight regain. This study contributes valuable insights into the management of post-bariatric weight regain.

Bibliography

1. Mok JKW, Makaronidis JM, Batterham RL. The role of gut hormones in obesity. Curr Opin Endocrine Metab Res. 2019; 4:4–13. This review summarizes the current knowledge on the role of gut hormones in the development and management of obesity.
2. Makaronidis JM, Batterham RL. The role of gut hormones in the pathogenesis and management of obesity. Curr Opin Physiol. 2019; 12:1–11. This review provides insights into the role of gut hormones as regulators of energy homeostasis, pathogenetic determinants of obesity and therapeutic targets for obesity treatment.
3. Berthoud HR. Metabolic and hedonic drives in the neural control of appetite: who is the boss? Curr Opin Neurobiol. 2011;21:888–96.
4. Monteiro MP, Batterham RL. The importance of the gastrointestinal tract in controlling food intake and regulating energy balance. Gastroenterology. 2017;152:1707–1717.e2.
5. Pilitsi E, Farr OM, Polyzos SA, Perakakis N, Nolen-Doerr E, Papathanasiou AE, et al. Pharmacotherapy of obesity: available medications and drugs under investigation. Metab Clin Exp. 2019; 92:170–92. This review summarizes the currently approved anti-obesity medication, and presents investigational agents in the pipeline for future therapeutic use, including pharmacotherapies targeting gut hormones.
6. Schwartz MW, Woods SC, Porte D Jr, Seeley RJ, Baskin DG. Central nervous system control of food intake. Nature. 2000;404:661–71.
7. Field BCT, Chaudhri OB, Bloom SR. Bowels control brain: gut hormones and obesity. Nat Rev Endocrinol. 2010;6:444–53.
8. Kojima M, Kangawa K. Ghrelin: structure and function. Physiol Rev. 2005;85:495–522.
9. De Silva A, Salem V, Long CJ, Makwana A, Newbould RD, Rabiner EA, et al. The gut hormones PYY 3-36 and GLP-1 7-36 amide reduce food intake and modulate brain activity in appetite centers in humans. Cell Metab. 2011;14:700–6.
10. Steinert RE, Feinle-Bisset C, Asarian L, Horowitz M, Beglinger C, Geary N. Ghrelin, CCK, GLP-1, and PYY(3–36): Secretory controls and physiological roles in eating and glycemia in health, obesity, and after RYGB. Physiol Rev. 2017;97:411–63. In this paper, the authors review the complex nutrient-sensing mechanisms that control the secretion of ghrelin, cholecystokinin (CCK), glucagon-like peptide-1 (GLP-1), and peptide tyrosine-tyrosine (PYY3-36) and summarize their contributions to the regulation of gastrointestinal function,

food intake and meal-related hyperglycaemia in normal-weight and obese subjects, as well as RYGB patients.
11. Adam TC, Westerterp-Plantenga MS. Glucagon-like peptide-1 release and satiety after a nutrient challenge in normal-weight and obese subjects. Br J Nutr. 2005;93:845–51.
12. Reda TK, Geliebter A, Pi-Sunyer FX. Amylin, food intake, and obesity. Obes Res. 2002;10:1087–91.
13. Dockray GJ. Cholecystokinin. Curr Opin Endocrinol Diabetes Obes. 2012;19:8–12.
14. Schmidt JB, Gregersen NT, Pedersen SD, Arentoft JL, Ritz C, Schwartz TW, et al. Effects of PYY3–36 and GLP-1 on energy intake, energy expenditure, and appetite in overweight men. Am J Physiol Endocrinol Metab. 2014;306:E1248–56.
15. Neary NM, Small CJ, Druce MRPAJ, Ellis SM, Semjonous NM, et al. Peptide YY3-36 and glucagon-like peptide-17-36 inhibit food intake additively. Endocrinology. 2005;146:5120–7.
16. Manning S, Batterham RL. The role of gut hormone peptide YY in energy and glucose homeostasis: twelve years on. Annu Rev Physiol. 2014;76:585–608.
17. Troke RC, Tan TM, Bloom SR. The future role of gut hormones in the treatment of obesity. Ther Adv Chronic Dis. 2014;5:4–14.
18. Trevaskis JL, Coffey T, Cole R, Lei C, Wittmer C, Walsh B, et al. Amylin-mediated restoration of leptin responsiveness in diet-induced obesity: magnitude and mechanisms. Endocrinology. 2008;149:5679–87.
19. Lean ME, Malkova D. Altered gut and adipose tissue hormones in overweight and obese individuals: cause or consequence? Int J Obes. 2016; 40:622–32. This review addresses the causality of the relationship between obesity and altered gut hormones and summarizes the major gut hormone modifications after weight loss with diet, exercise and bariatric surgery, which may be relevant for future obesity treatment strategies.
20. Kokkinos A, Tsilingiris D, le Roux CW, Rubino F, Mantzoros CS. Will medications that mimic gut hormones or target their receptors eventually replace bariatric surgery? Metabolism. 2019;100:153960. This paper reviews current evidence regarding the gut peptides' physiology and their role in weight loss after bariatric surgery, along with the evolving aspects in the field of gut peptide-based obesity and T2DM therapies.
21. Wölnerhanssen BK, Moran AW, Burdyga G, Meyer-Gerspach AC, Peterli R, Manz M, et al. Deregulation of transcription factors controlling intestinal epithelial cell differentiation; a predisposing factor for reduced enteroendocrine cell number in morbidly obese individuals. Sci Rep. 2017;7:8174. This study is important because it provides an explanation for the impaired gut hormone secretion of morbidly obese individuals. The authors propose that morbid obesity is associated with a dysregulated differentiation of intestinal epithelial cells that may influence the levels of released gut hormones. Interestingly, this aberrant cellular differentiation profile is restored after bariatric surgery (sleeve gastrectomy).
22. Mishra AK, Dubey V, Ghosh AR. Obesity: an overview of possible role(s) of gut hormones, lipid sensing and gut microbiota. Metabolism. 2016;65:48–65.
23. Cummings DE, Weigle DS, Frayo RS, Breen PA, Ma MK, Dellinger EP, et al. Plasma ghrelin levels after diet-induced weight loss or gastric bypass surgery. N Engl J Med. 2002;346:1623–30.
24. Zhao X, Han Q, Gang X, Lv Y, Liu Y, Sun C, et al. The role of gut hormones in diet-induced weight change: a systematic review. Horm Metab Res. 2017;49:816–25.
25. Crujeiras AB, Goyenechea E, Abete I, Lage M, Carreira MC, Martínez JA, et al. Weight regain after a diet-induced loss is predicted by higher baseline leptin and lower ghrelin plasma levels. J Clin Endocrinol Metab. 2010;95:5037–44.
26. Nymo S, Coutinho SR, Eknes PH, Vestbostad I, Rehfeld JF, Truby H, et al. Investigation of the long-term sustainability of changes in appetite after weight loss. Int J Obes. 2018;42:1489–99.
27. King JA, Wasse LK, Ewens J, Crystallis K, Emmanuel J, Batterham RL, et al. Differential acylated ghrelin, peptide YY3–36, appetite, and food intake responses to equivalent energy deficits created by exercise and food restriction. J Clin Endocrinol Metab. 2011;96:1114–21.

28. Deighton K, Barry R, Connon CE, Stensel DJ. Appetite, gut hormone and energy intake responses to low volume sprint interval and traditional endurance exercise. Eur J Appl Physiol. 2013;113:1147–56.
29. Jones TE, Basilio JL, Brophy PM, McCammon MR, Hickner RC. Long-term exercise training in overweight adolescents improves plasma peptide YY and resistin. Obesity (Silver Spring). 2009;17:1189–95.
30. Perakakis N, Kokkinos A, Peradze N, Tentolouris N, Ghaly W, Pilitsi E, et al. Circulating levels of gastrointestinal hormones in response to the most common types of bariatric surgery and predictive value for weight loss over one year: evidence from two independent trials. Metabolism. 2019;101:153997. This study aimed to investigate the changes of circulating gastrointestinal hormones in response to the most common types of bariatric surgery and whether these changes can predict future weight loss. The authors reported that beyond GLP-1, early postprandial changes in circulating oxyntomodulin and glicentin levels are strong predictors of prospective weight loss after surgery, possibly through regulation of satiety.
31. Field BC, Wren AM, Peters V, Baynes KC, Martin NM, Patterson M, et al. PYY3-36 and oxyntomodulin can be additive in their effect on food intake in overweight and obese humans. Diabetes. 2010;59:1635–9.
32. World Health Organization. Obesity and overweight: fact sheet no. 311. 2014. http://www.who.int/mediacentre/factsheets/fs311/en/. Accessed 22 Jan 2015.
33. Angulo P. Nonalcoholic fatty liver disease. N Engl J Med. 2002;346(16):1221–31.
34. Bray GA. Why do we need drugs to treat the patient with obesity? Obesity. 2013;21(5):893–9.
35. Jensen MD, Ryan DH, Apovian CM, Ard JD, Comuzzie AG, Donato KA, et al. AHA/ACC/TOS guideline for the management of overweight and obesity in adults: a report of the American College of Cardiology/American Heart Association Task Force on Practice Guidelines and the Obesity Society. J Am Coll Cardiol. 2013;63(25 Pt B):2985–3023.
36. Wright F, Boyle S, Baxter K, et al. Understanding the relationship between weight loss, emotional well-being and health-related quality of life in patients attending a specialist obesity weight management service. J Health Psychol. 2013;18(4):574–86.
37. Kuna ST, Reboussin DM, Borradaile KE, et al. Long-term effect of weight loss on obstructive sleep apnea severity in obese patients with type 2 diabetes. Sleep. 2013;36(5):641–9.
38. Scott LJ. Liraglutide: a review of its use in patients with type 2 diabetes mellitus. Drugs. 2014;74(18):2161–74.
39. Horowitz M, Flint A, Jones KL, et al. Effect of the once-daily human GLP-1 analogue liraglutide on appetite, energy intake, energy expenditure and gastric emptying in type 2 diabetes. Diabetes Res Clin Pract. 2012;97(2):258–66.
40. Fujishima Y, Maeda N, Inoue K, et al. Efficacy of liraglutide, a glucagon-like peptide-1 (GLP-1) analogue, on body weight, eating behavior, and glycemic control, in Japanese obese type 2 diabetes. Cardiovasc Diabetol. 2012;11:107.
41. Van Can J, Sloth B, Jensen CB, et al. Effects of the once-daily GLP-1 analog liraglutide on gastric emptying, glycemic parameters, appetite and energy metabolism in obese, non-diabetic adults. Int J Obes. 2014;38(6):784–93.
42. Jendle J, Nauck MA, Matthews DR, et al. Weight loss with liraglutide, a once-daily human glucagon-like peptide-1 analogue for type 2 diabetes treatment as monotherapy or added to metformin, is primarily as a result of a reduction in fat tissue. Antimicrob Agents Chemother. 2009;11(12):1163–72.
43. Novo Nordisk. Saxenda® liragluitde (rDNA) injection: US prescribing information. 2014. http://www.saxenda.com/ . Accessed 21 Jan 2014.
44. European Medicines Agency. Saxenda: summary of product characteristics. 2015. http://ec.europa.eu/health/documents/community-register/html/h992.htm#EndOfPage. Accessed 26 Mar 2015.

45. Wadden TA, Hollander P, Klein S, Niswender K, Woo V, Hale PM, et al. Weight maintenance and additional weight loss with liraglutide after low-calorie-diet-induced weight loss: the SCALE maintenance randomized study. Int J Obes. 2013;37(11):1443–51.
46. Bode B, DeFronzo R, Bergenstal R, et al. Effect of liraglutide 3.0/1.8 mg on body weight and cardiometabolic risk factors in overweight/obese adults with type 2 diabetes: SCALE Diabetes randomised, double-blind, 56-week trial [abstract no. 181]. Diabetologia. 2014;57(1 Suppl 1):S83.
47. Egan AG, Blind E, Dunder K, de Graeff PA, Hummer BT, Bourcier T, et al. Pancreatic safety of incretin-based drugs—FDA and EMA assessment. N Engl J Med. 2014;370(9):794–7.
48. Womble LG, Wadden TA, Chandler JM, Martin AR. Agreement between weekly vs. daily assessment of appetite. Appetite. 2003;40:131–5.
49. Sorli C, Harashima SI, Tsoukas GM, et al. Efficacy and safety of once-weekly semaglutide monotherapy versus placebo in patients with type 2 diabetes (SUSTAIN 1): a double-blind, randomised, placebo-controlled, parallel-group, multinational, multicentre phase 3a trial. Lancet Diabetes Endocrinol. 2017;5(4):251–60.
50. Marso SP, Bain SC, Consoli A, et al. Semaglutide and cardiovascular outcomes in patients with type 2 diabetes. N Engl J Med. 2016;375(19):1834–44.
51. R.F. Kushner, S. Calanna, M. Davies et al. Semaglutide 2.4 mg for the treatment of obesity: key elements of the STEP trials 1 to 5. Obes. (Silver Spring) 28(6), 1050–1061 (2020).
52. Davies M, Færch L, Jeppesen OK, et al. Semaglutide 2·4 mg once a week in adults with overweight or obesity, and type 2 diabetes (STEP 2): a randomised, double-blind, double-dummy, placebo-controlled, phase 3 trial. Lancet. 2021;397(10278):971–84.
53. Jensen MD, et al. 2013 AHA/ACC/TOS guideline for the management of overweight and obesity in adults: a report of the American College of Cardiology/American Heart Association Task Force on Practice Guidelines and The Obesity Society. Circulation. 2014;129:S102–38.
54. Wegovy prescribing information. Updated June 2021. US Food and Drug Administration https://www.accessdata.fda.gov/drugsatfda_docs/label/2021/215256s000lbl.pdf (2022).
55. Wegovy summary of product characteristics. European Medicines Agency https://www.ema.europa.eu/en/documents/product-information/wegovy-epar-product-information_en.pdf (2022).
56. Regulatory decision summary—Wegovy. Health Canada. https://hpr-rps.hres.ca/reg-content/regulatory-decision-summary-detail.php?lang=en&linkID=RDS00896 (2022).
57. Wegovy summary of product characteristics. Medicines and Healthcare Products Regulatory Agency https://mhraproducts4853.blob.core.windows.net/docs/ee95471f9265e346688fce45e8c9fd8bd5e4e3d3 (2022).
58. Wilding JPH, Batterham RL, Calanna S, et al. Once-weekly semaglutide in adults with overweight or obesity. N Engl J Med. 2021;384(11):989–1002.
59. Wadden TA, Bailey TS, Billings LK, et al. Effect of subcutaneous semaglutide vs placebo as an adjunct to intensive behavioral therapy on body weight in adults with overweight or obesity: the STEP 3 randomized clinical trial. JAMA. 2021;325(14):1403–13.
60. Obokata M, Reddy YNV, Pislaru SV, Melenovsky V, Borlaug BA. Evidence supporting the existence of a distinct obese phenotype of heart failure with preserved ejection fraction. Circulation. 2017;136:6–19.
61. Reddy YNV, et al. Characterization of the obese phenotype of heart failure with preserved ejection fraction: a RELAX trial ancillary study. Mayo Clin Proc. 2019;94:1199–209.
62. Reddy YNV, et al. Quality of life in heart failure with preserved ejection fraction: importance of obesity, functional capacity, and physical inactivity. Eur J Heart Fail. 2020;22:1009–18.
63. Kitzman DW, et al. Effect of caloric restriction or aerobic exercise training on peak oxygen consumption and quality of life in obese older patients with heart failure with preserved ejection fraction: a randomized clinical trial. JAMA. 2016;315:36–46.
64. American Diabetes Association Professional Practice Committee, Draznin B, Aroda VR, Bakris G, Benson G, Brown FM, et al. 8. Obesity and weight management for the prevention

and treatment of Type 2 Diabetes: Standards of Medical Care in Diabetes-2022. Diabetes Care 2022;45:S113–S124.

65. Min T, Bain SC. The Role of Tirzepatide, Dual GIP and GLP-1 Receptor Agonist, in the Management of Type 2 Diabetes: The SURPASS Clinical Trials. Diabetes Ther. 2021;12:143–57.
66. Coskun T, Sloop KW, Loghin C, Alsina-Fernandez J, Urva S, Bokvist KB, et al. LY3298176, a novel dual GIP and GLP-1 receptor agonist for the treatment of type 2 diabetes mellitus: from discovery to clinical proof of concept. Mol Metab. 2018;18:3–14.
67. Chavda VP, Ajabiya J, Teli D, Bojarska J, Apostolopoulos V. Tirzepatide, a new era of dual-targeted treatment for diabetes and obesity: a mini-review. Molecules. 2022;27:4315.
68. Schünemann H, Brożek J, Guyatt G, Oxman A GRADE handbook for grading quality of evidence and strength of recommendations. 2013. https://gdt.gradepro.org/app/handbook/handbook.html
69. Jastreboff AM, Aronne LJ, Ahmad NN, Wharton S, Connery L, Alves B, et al. Tirzepatide once weekly for the treatment of obesity. N Engl J Med. 2022;387:205–16.
70. Rosenstock J, Wysham C, Frías JP, Kaneko S, Lee CJ, Fernández Landó L, et al. Efficacy and safety of a novel dual GIP and GLP-1 receptor agonist tirzepatide in patients with type 2 diabetes (SURPASS-1): a double-blind, randomised, phase 3 trial [published correction appears in Lancet. 2021 Jul 17; 398(10296):212]. Lancet. 2021;398:143–55.
71. Dahl D, Onishi Y, Norwood P, Huh R, Bray R, Patel H, et al. Effect of subcutaneous Tirzepatide vs placebo added to titrated insulin glargine on glycemic control in patients with type 2 diabetes: the SURPASS-5 randomized clinical trial. JAMA. 2022;327:534–45.
72. Del Prato S, Kahn SE, Pavo I, Weerakkody GJ, Yang Z, Doupis J, et al. Tirzepatide versus insulin glargine in type 2 diabetes and increased cardiovascular risk (SURPASS-4): a randomised, open-label, parallel-group, multicentre, phase 3 trial. Lancet. 2021;398:1811–24.
73. Frías JP, Davies MJ, Rosenstock J, Pérez Manghi FC, Fernández Landó L, Bergman BK, et al. Tirzepatide versus Semaglutide once weekly in patients with type 2 diabetes. N Engl J Med. 2021;385:503–15.
74. Page MJ, McKenzie JE, Bossuyt PM, Boutron I, Hoffmann TC, Mulrow CD, et al. The PRISMA 2020 statement: an updated guideline for reporting systematic reviews. BMJ. 2021;372:n71.
75. Karagiannis T, Avgerinos I, Liakos A, Del Prato S, Matthews DR, Tsapas A, et al. Management of type 2 diabetes with the dual GIP/GLP-1 receptor agonist tirzepatide: a systematic review and meta-analysis. Diabetologia. 2022;65:1251–61.
76. Bhagavathula AS, Vidyasagar K, Tesfaye W. Efficacy and safety of Tirzepatide in patients with type 2 diabetes mellitus: a systematic review and meta-analysis of randomized phase II/III trials. Pharmaceuticals (Basel). 2021;14:991.
77. Jung HN, Jung CH. The upcoming weekly tides (Semaglutide vs. Tirzepatide) against obesity: STEP or SURPASS? Review. J Obes Metab Syndr. 2022;31:28–36. https://doi.org/10.7570/JOMES22012.
78. Vosoughi K, Atieh J, Khanna L, Khoshbin K, Prokop LJ, Davitkov P, et al. Association of glucagon-like peptide 1 analogs and agonists administered for obesity with weight loss and adverse events: a systematic review and network meta-analysis. EClinicalMedicine. 2021;42:101213. https://doi.org/10.1016/j.eclinm.2021.101213.
79. Cacciottolo TM, Evans K. Research in brief: effective pharmacotherapy for the management of obesity. Clin Med (Lond). 2021;21:e517–8. https://doi.org/10.7861/clinmed.2021-0253.
80. Fornes A, Huff J, Pritchard RI, Godfrey M. Once-weekly semaglutide for weight management: a clinical review. J Pharm Technol. 2022;38:239–46. https://doi.org/10.1177/87551225221092681.
81. Ng CH, Lin SY, Chin YH, Lee MH, Syn N, Goh XL, et al. Antidiabetic medications for type 2 diabetics with nonalcoholic fatty liver disease: evidence from a network meta-analysis of randomized controlled trials. Endocr Pract. 2022;28:223–30. https://doi.org/10.1016/j.eprac.2021.09.013.

82. Quek J, Chan KE, Wong ZY, Tan C, Tan B, Lim WH, et al. Global prevalence of non-alcoholic fatty liver disease and non-alcoholic steatohepatitis in the overweight and obese population: a systematic review and meta-analysis. Lancet Gastroenterol Hepatol. 2023;8:20–30. https://doi.org/10.1016/s2468-1253(22)00317-x.
83. Roborel de Climens A, Pain E, Boss A, Shaunik A. Understanding reasons for treatment discontinuation, attitudes and education needs among people who discontinue type 2 diabetes treatment: results from an online patient survey in the USA and UK. Diabetes Ther. 2020;11:1873–81. https://doi.org/10.1007/s13300-020-00843-9.
84. Pi-Sunyer X, Astrup A, Fujioka K, Greenway F, Halpern A, Krempf M, et al. A randomized, controlled trial of 3.0 mg of liraglutide in weight management. N Engl J Med. 2015;373:11–22.
85. le Roux CW, Astrup A, Fujioka K, Greenway F, Lau DCW, Van Gaal L, Ortiz RV, Wilding JPH, Skjøth TV, Manning LS, Pi-Sunyer X, SCALE Obesity Prediabetes NN8022-1839 Study Group. 3 years of liraglutide versus placebo for type 2 diabetes risk reduction and weight management in individuals with prediabetes: a randomised, double-blind trial. Lancet. 2017;389:1399–409. https://doi.org/10.1016/S0140-6736(17)30069-7.
86. Davies MJ, et al. Efficacy of liraglutide for weight loss among patients with type 2 diabetes: the SCALE diabetes randomized clinical trial. JAMA. 2015;314:687–99.
87. Wadden TA, Walsh OA, Berkowitz RI, Chao AM, Alamuddin N, Gruber K, et al. Intensive behavioral therapy for obesity combined with liraglutide 3.0 mg: a randomized controlled trial. Obesity (Silver Spring). 2019;27:75–86.
88. Rubino D, Abrahamsson N, Davies M, et al. Effect of continued weekly subcutaneous Semaglutide vs Placebo on weight loss maintenance in adults with overweight or obesity: the STEP 4 randomized clinical trial. JAMA. 2021;325(14):1414–25.
89. Garvey WT, Batterham RL, Bhatta M, Buscemi S, Christensen LN, Frias JP, et al. Two-year effects of semaglutide in adults with overweight or obesity: the STEP 5 trial. Nat Med. 2022;28:2083–91.
90. Kadowaki T, Isendahl J, Khalid U, Lee SY, Nishida T, Ogawa W, et al. Semaglutide once a week in adults with overweight or obesity, with or without type 2 diabetes in an east Asian population (STEP 6): a randomised, double-blind, double-dummy, placebo-controlled, phase 3a trial. Lancet Diabetes Endocrinol. 2022;10:193–206.
91. Rubino DM, et al. STEP 8 Investigators. Effect of weekly subcutaneous semaglutide vs daily liraglutide on body weight in adults with overweight or obesity without diabetes: the STEP 8 randomized clinical trial. JAMA. 2022;327:138–50.
92. Garvey WT, Frias JP, Jastreboff AM, le Roux CW, Sattar N, Aizenberg D, et al. Tirzepatide once weekly for the treatment of obesity in people with type 2 diabetes (SURMOUNT-2): a double-blind, randomised, multicentre, placebo-controlled, phase 3 trial. Lancet. 2023;402:613–26.
93. Wadden TA, Chao AM, Machineni S, Kushner R, Ard J, Srivastava G, et al. Tirzepatide after intensive lifestyle intervention in adults with overweight or obesity: the SURMOUNT-3 phase 3 trial. Nat Med. 2023;29:2909–18. https://doi.org/10.1038/s41591-023-02597-w.
94. Aronne LJ, Sattar N, Horn DB, Bays HE, Wharton S, Lin WY, et al. Tirze weight maintenance. Continued treatment with tirzepatide for maintenance of weight reduction in adults with obesity: the SURMOUNT-4 randomized clinical trial. JAMA. 2024;331:38–48.
95. Lincoff AM, Brown-Frandsen K, Colhoun HM, Deanfield J, Emerson SS, Esbjerg S, et al. Semaglutide and cardiovascular outcomes in obesity without diabetes. N Engl J Med. 2023;389:2221–32.
96. Htike ZZ, Zaccardi F, Papamargaritis D, Webb DR, Khunti K, Davies MJ. Efficacy and safety of glucagon-like peptide-1 receptor agonists in type 2 diabetes: a systematic review and mixed-treatment comparison analysis. Diabetes Obes Metab. 2017;19(4):524–36.
97. Newsome NP, Buchholtz K, Cusi K, Linder M, Okanoue T, Ratziu V, et al. A placebo-controlled trial of subcutaneous semaglutide in nonalcoholic steatohepatitis. N Engl J Med. 2021;384:1113–24.

98. ClinicalTrials.gov. A research study to look at how semaglutide compared to placebo affects diabetic eye disease in people with type 2 diabetes (FOCUS). 2023. https://clinicaltrials.gov/ct2/show/NCT03811561
99. Marso SP, Daniels GH, Brown-Frandsen K, Kristensen P, Mann JF, Nauck MA, et al. Liraglutide and cardiovascular outcomes in type 2 diabetes. N Engl J Med. 2016;375:311–22.
100. Leehey DJ, Rahman MA, Borys E, Picken MM, Clise CE. Acute kidney injury associated with semaglutide. Kidney Med. 2021;3:282–5.
101. Heerspink HJL, Apperloo E, Davies M, Dicker D, Kandler K, Rosenstock J, et al. Effects of semaglutide on albuminuria and kidney function in people with overweight or obesity with or without type 2 diabetes: exploratory analysis from the STEP 1, 2, and 3 trials. Diabetes Care. 2023;46:801–10.
102. Nauck MA, Friedrich N. Do GLP-1-based therapies increase cancer risk? Diabetes Care. 2013;36:S245–52.
103. Bezin J, Gouverneur A, Pénichon M, Mathieu C, Garrel R, Hillaire-Buys D, et al. GLP-1 receptor agonists and the risk of thyroid cancer. Diabetes Care. 2023;46:384–90.
104. Mali G, Ahuja V, Dubey K. Glucagon-like peptide-1 analogues and thyroid cancer: an analysis of cases reported in the European pharmacovigilance database. J Clin Pharm Ther. 2021;46:99–105.
105. Pradhan R, Patorno E, Tesfaye H, Schneeweiss S, Yin H, Franklin J, et al. Glucagon-like peptide 1 receptor agonists and risk of anaphylactic reaction among patients with type 2 diabetes: a multisite population-based cohort study. Am J Epidemiol. 2022;191:1352–67.
106. Jacobsen LV, Vouis J, Hindsberger C, Zdravkovic M. Treatment with liraglutide–a once-daily GLP-1 analog–does not reduce the bioavailability of ethinyl estradiol/levonorgestrel taken as an oral combination contraceptive drug. J Clin Pharmacol. 2011;51:1696–703.
107. Kapitza C, Nosek L, Jensen L, Hartvig H, Jensen CB, Flint A. Semaglutide, a once-weekly human GLP-1 analog, does not reduce the bioavailability of the combined oral contraceptive, ethinylestradiol/levonorgestrel. J Clin Pharmacol. 2015;55:497–504.
108. Schultes B, Ernst B, Timper K, Puder J, Rudofsky G. Pharmacological interventions for weight loss before conception-putative effects on subsequent gestational weight gain should be considered. Int J Obes. 2023;47:335–7.
109. Nuako A, Tu L, Reyes KJC, Chhabria SM, Stanford FC. Pharmacologic treatment of obesity in reproductive aged women. Curr Obstet Gynecol Rep. 2023;12:138–46.
110. Muller DRP, Stenvers DJ, Malekzadeh A, Holleman F, Painter RC, Siegelaar SE. Effects of GLP-1 agonists and SGLT2 inhibitors during pregnancy and lactation on offspring outcomes: a systematic review of the evidence. Front Endocrinol (Lausanne). 2023;14:1215356.
111. Cesta CE, Rotem R, Bateman BT, Chodick G, Cohen JM, Furu K, et al. Safety of GLP-1 receptor agonists and other second-line antidiabetics in early pregnancy. JAMA Intern Med. 2024;184:144–52.
112. Sodhi M, Rezaeianzadeh R, Kezouh A, Etminan M. Risk of gastrointestinal adverse events associated with glucagon-like peptide-1 receptor agonists for weight loss. JAMA. 2023;5:e2319574.
113. Fountoulakis KN, Gonda X, Baghai TC, Baldwin DS, Bauer M, Blier P, et al. Report of the WPA section of pharmacopsychiatry on the relationship of antiepileptic drugs with suicidality in epilepsy. Int J Psychiatry Clin Pract. 2015;19:158–67.
114. Lautenbach A, Wernecke M, Huber TB, et al. The potential of semaglutide once-weekly in patients without type 2 diabetes with weight regain or insufficient weight loss after bariatric surgery—a retrospective analysis. Obes Surg. 2022;32(10):3280–8.
115. Rothkopf MM, Bilof ML, Haverstick LP, Nusbaum MJ. Synergistic weight loss and diabetes resolution with exenatide administration after laparoscopic gastric banding. Surg Obes Relat Dis. 2009;5(1):128–31.
116. Pajecki D, Halpern A, Cercato C, Mancini M, de Cleva R, Santo MA. Tratamento de curto prazo com liraglutide no reganho de peso após cirurgia bariátrica. Rev Colégio Bras Cir. 2013;40(3):191–5.

117. Gorgojo-Martínez JJ, Feo-Ortega G, Serrano-Moreno C. Effectiveness and tolerability of liraglutide in patients with type 2 diabetes mellitus and obesity after bariatric surgery. Surg Obes Relat Dis. 2016;12(10):1856–63.
118. Creange C, Lin E, Ren-Fielding C, Lofton H. Use of liraglutide for weight loss in patients with prior bariatric surgery. Surg Obes Relat Dis. 2016;12(7):S157.
119. Rye P, Modi R, Cawsey S, Sharma AM. Efficacy of high-dose liraglutide as an adjunct for weight loss in patients with prior bariatric surgery. Obes Surg. 2018;28(11):3553–8.
120. Wharton S, Kuk JL, Luszczynski M, et al. Liraglutide 3.0 mg for the management of insufficient weight loss or excessive weight regain post-bariatric surgery. Clin Obes. 2019;9(4):e12323.
121. Suliman M, Buckley A, Al Tikriti A, Tan T, le Roux CW, Lessan N, Barakat M. Routine clinical use of liraglutide 3 mg for the treatment of obesity: outcomes in non-surgical and bariatric surgery patients. Diabetes Obes Metab. 2019;21(6):1498–501.
122. Bretault M, Carette C, Zaharia R, Vychnevskaia K, Bouillot JL, Czernichow S, Raffin-Sanson ML. Liraglutide 3 mg as a weight-loss strategy after failed bariatric surgery in a patient with hypothalamic obesity following craniopharyngioma. Diabetes Metab. 2020;46(6):514–5.
123. Rubio MA, Ramos-Leví AM. Initial experience with alternate-day liraglutide for weight regain following bariatric surgery. Obes Surg. 2021;31(9):4216–8.
124. Horber FF, Steffen R. Reversal of long-term weight regain after Roux-en-Y gastric bypass using liraglutide or surgical revision. A prospective study. Obes Surg. 2021;31(1):93–100.
125. Elhag W, El Ansari W. Effectiveness and safety of liraglutide in managing inadequate weight loss and weight regain after primary and revisional bariatric surgery: anthropometric and cardiometabolic outcomes. Obes Surg. 2022;32(4):1005–15.
126. Dharmaratnam VM, Lim E, Eng A, et al. Revisional surgery or pharmacotherapy for insufficient weight loss and weight regain after primary bariatric procedure: a descriptive study. Obes Surg. 2022;32(10):3298–304.
127. Rubino DM, Greenway FL, Khalid U, O'Neil PM, Rosenstock J, Sørrig R, Wadden TA, Wizert A, Garvey WT, STEP 8 Investigators, Arauz-Pacheco C, Cannon K, Downey HJ, Fitz-Patrick D, Geohas J, Gerety G, Gilbert J, Hollander P, Klein E, Laufer K, O'Donnell P, Rosenblit P, Toth P. Effect of weekly subcutaneous semaglutide vs daily liraglutide on body weight in adults with overweight or obesity without diabetes: the STEP 8 randomized clinical trial. JAMA. 2022;327(2):138.
128. Koliaki C, Liatis S, Dalamaga M, Kokkinos A. The implication of gut hormones in the regulation of energy homeostasis and their role in the pathophysiology of obesity. Curr Obes Rep. 2020;9:255–71. https://doi.org/10.1007/s13679-020-00396-9.
129. Scott LJ. Liraglutide: a review of its use in the management of obesity. Drugs. 2015;75:899–910. https://doi.org/10.1007/s40265-015-0408-8.
130. Tronieri JS, Wadden TA, Walsh, Olivia; Berkowitz, Robert I.; Alamuddin, Naji; Gruber, Kathryn; Leonard, Sharon; Bakizada, Zayna M.; Chao, Ariana M. Effects of liraglutide on appetite, food preoccupation, and food liking: results of a randomized controlled trial. Int J Obes. 2019;44:353–61. https://doi.org/10.1038/s41366-019-0348-6.
131. Zhong P, Zeng H, Huang M, Fu W, Chen Z. Efficacy and safety of once-weekly semaglutide in adults with overweight or obesity: a meta-analysis. Endocrine. 2022;75:718–24. https://doi.org/10.1007/s12020-021-02945-1.
132. Garvey WT, Batterham RL, Bhatta M, Buscemi S, Christensen LN, Frias JP, Jódar E, Kandler K, Rigas G, Wadden TA, Wharton S. Two-year effects of semaglutide in adults with overweight or obesity: the STEP 5 trial. Nat Med. 2022;28:2083–91. https://doi.org/10.1038/s41591-022-02026-4.
133. Borlaug BA, Kitzman DW, Davies MJ, Rasmussen S, Barros E, Butler J, Einfeldt MN, Hovingh GK, Møller DV, Petrie MC, Shah SJ, Verma S, Abhayaratna W, Ahmed FZ, Chopra V, Ezekowitz J, Fu M, Ito H, Lelonek M, Melenovsky V, Núñez J, Perna E, Schou M, Senni M, van der Meer P, Von Lewinski D, Wolf D, Kosiborod MN. Semaglutide in HFpEF across obesity class and by body weight reduction: a prespecified analysis of the STEP-HFpEF trial. Nat Med. 2023;29:2358–65. https://doi.org/10.1038/s41591-023-02526-x.

134. de Mesquita YLL, Pera Calvi I, Reis Marques I, Almeida Cruz S, Padrao EMH, Carvalho PEDP, da Silva CHA, Cardoso R, Moura FA, Rafalskiy VV. Efficacy and safety of the dual GIP and GLP-1 receptor agonist tirzepatide for weight loss: a meta-analysis of randomized controlled trials. Int J Obes. 2023;47:883–92. https://doi.org/10.1038/s41366-023-01337-x.
135. Tan B, Pan X-H, Chew HSJ, Goh RSJ, Lin C, Anand VV, Lee ECZ, Chan KE, Kong G, Ong CEY, Chung HC, Young DY, Chan MY, Khoo CM, Mehta A, Muthiah MD, Noureddin M, Ng CH, Chew NWS, Chin YH. Efficacy and safety of tirzepatide for treatment of overweight or obesity. A systematic review and meta-analysis. Int J Obes. 2023;47:677–85. https://doi.org/10.1038/s41366-023-01321-5.
136. Vidal J, Flores L, Jiménez A, Pané A, de Hollanda A. What is the evidence regarding the safety of new obesity pharmacotherapies. Int J Obes. 2024; https://doi.org/10.1038/s41366-024-01488-5.
137. Jensen AB, Renström F, Aczél S, Folie P, Biraima-Steinemann M, Beuschlein F, Bilz S. Efficacy of the glucagon-like peptide-1 receptor agonists Liraglutide and Semaglutide for the treatment of weight regain after bariatric surgery: a retrospective observational study. Obes Surg. 2023;33:1017–25. https://doi.org/10.1007/s11695-023-06484-8.

Chapter 5
Anti-obesity Medications for Monogenic Syndromic Obesity

Shilpa Chugh Garcha and Sanjay Kalra

Obesity generally occurs due to an interplay of two important factors: genetic and environmental and basis these factors, it can be broadly classified into polygenic obesity and monogenic obesity. Monogenic obesity is the basis for rare obesity syndromes.

Melanocortin-4 receptor (MC4R) agonists are promising treatment options for the management of monogenic obesity. MC4R pathway is a key regulator of hunger, satiety, and energy balance, and impaired MC4R pathway signaling is suggested to result in hyperphagia and decreased energy expenditure which leads to obesity.

Studies have been included in this chapter on the role of MC4R agonist Setmelanotide in the management of monogenic obesity syndromes: Bardet–Biedl syndrome (BBS), Alström syndrome, and Prader–Willi syndrome.

Setmelanotide is an MC4R agonist that is USFDA-approved for patients 6 years of age and older, for chronic weight management in people with obesity due to pro-opiomelanocortin (POMC), proprotein convertase subtilisin/kexin type 1 (PCSK1) or leptin receptor deficiency (LEPR), confirmed by genetic testing that demonstrates variants in these genes which are interpreted as pathogenic, likely pathogenic, or of uncertain significance (VUS) [1]. It is available as a subcutaneous injectable formulation.

Two studies exploring the role and impact of Setmelanotide on BBS have been included in this chapter. BBS is a rare genetic syndrome with impaired signaling in the MC4R pathway marked by obesity, hyperphagia, primary dysfunction of cilia, and multiorgan failure. One of the studies in patients with BBS delves into the impact of the setmelanotide on health-related quality of life (HRQOL) in these patients. After one year of treatment, clinically significant reductions in body weight

S. C. Garcha (✉)
Sonepat, Haryana, India

S. Kalra
Department of Endocrinology, Bharti Hospital, Karnal, Haryana, India

S. C. Garcha, S. Kalra (eds.), *Drugs for Medical Management of Obesity*,
https://doi.org/10.1007/978-981-96-1651-0_5

and hunger scores were seen. This study highlighted the potential of setmelanotide in improving physical function, psychological well-being, and improving HRQOL.

One study exploring two case reports of individuals with compound heterozygous leptin receptor deficiency and currently on setmelanotide has been included. This study underscores the importance of early genetic screening for patients with hyperphagia and early onset obesity as lifestyle modifications, behavioral therapies and even evidence for efficacy of bariatric surgery is limited. The study highlights that although there is an increasing awareness about the genetic impact on obesity, early identification, and diagnosis of the condition remain challenging.

Metreleptin

Lipodystrophy syndromes are rare medical conditions (genetic or acquired), characterized by tissue deficiency in some areas and excessive lipid deposition in unaffected areas.

Metreleptin, a recombinant analog of the human hormone leptin is indicated as an adjunct to diet as replacement therapy to treat leptin deficiency complications in patients with congenital or acquired generalized lipodystrophy [2]. It is a subcutaneous formulation and is the only medication available as a specific treatment for lipodystrophy.

One of the studies included explores the role of metreleptin in the management of lipodystrophies. Metreleptin binds to the leptin receptors and mimics the physiological effects of leptin including regulation of appetite and metabolic parameters. This study also focuses on the tolerability of metreleptin stating that although metreleptin is well tolerable and has an adverse effect profile similar across ages, however, there are concerns regarding its potential for immunogenicity, pancreatitis, and T cell lymphoma.

Other Anti-Obesity Medications for Syndromic Obesity

One of the studies included in this chapter explores the role of various available anti-obesity medications in the management of obesity syndrome, Prader-willi syndrome.

Prader-willi syndrome is a genetic disorder characterized by hyperphagia, morbid obesity with an increased risk of type 2 diabetes and obstructive sleep apnoea, intellectual impairment, and short stature. This study provided a real-world view of the effect of very-low energy diets (VLEDs) given along with pharmacotherapies including phentermine-topiramate or naltrexone-bupropion or liraglutide in the management of Prader-willi syndrome. Even though most of the patients achieved clinically effective weight loss; non-adherence and discontinuation due to adverse effects in the patients taking phentermine-topiramate was an important concern.

To summarise, newer medications that are effective and tolerable are becoming available for the management of monogenic syndromic obesity, however, lack of awareness and delayed diagnosis of these patients remain challenging. More case reports and clinical studies are needed to explore the role of these medications in real-world scenarios and a better understanding of their use. More studies are also needed to explore the efficacy and tolerability of drugs available for non-syndromic obesity in the management of monogenic syndromic obesity.

References for Introduction

(1) IMCIVREE® (Setmelanotide) injection U.S. Food and Drug Administration website. https://www.accessdata.fda.gov/drugsatfda_docs/label/2022/213793s001lbl.pdf Revised Jun 2022. Accessed 8 Aug 2024

(2) MYALEPT (metreleptin). U.S. Food and Drug Administration website. https://www.accessdata.fda.gov/drugsatfda_docs/label/2014/125390s004lbl.pdf Revised Jun 2014. Accessed 14 Aug 2024

5.1 Machine Generated Summaries

Disclaimer: The summaries in this chapter were generated from Springer Nature publications using abstractive AI auto-summarization: An abstraction-based summarizer creates new text based on deep learning. New phrases are created to summarize the content. As the constituted sentences are machine selected, they may not fully reflect the body of the work, so we strongly advise that the original content is read and cited. The auto-generated summaries were curated by the editor to meet Springer Nature publication standards.

Machine generated keywords: setmelanotide, hyperphagia, mcr, lepr, leptin, leptin receptor, pomc.

The Promise of New Anti-obesity Therapies Arising from Knowledge of Genetic Obesity Traits [99]

This is a machine-generated summary of:

Hinney, Anke; Körner, Antje; Fischer-Posovszky, Pamela: The promise of new anti-obesity therapies arising from knowledge of genetic obesity traits [99].

Published in: Nature Reviews Endocrinology (2022)

Link to original: https://doi.org/10.1038/s41574-022-00716-0

If you want to cite the papers, please refer to the original.

For technical reasons we could not place the page where the original quote is coming from.

Research highlights

Introduction:

The global obesity epidemic has reached alarming proportions, with the World Health Organization reporting approximately 39 million children under five years age suffering from overweight or obesity. The early onset of obesity is closely associated with the development of cardiovascular and metabolic comorbidities, leading to increased mortality in adulthood. While common childhood obesity results from a mix of genetic predisposition and environmental factors, the COVID-19 pandemic has exacerbated the situation, highlighting the vulnerability of children with existing obesity to further weight gain during lockdowns. Now a new study by Anke Hinney and colleagues delves into the heritability of body weight and genetic classifications of obesity, discussing clinical features of early-onset monogenic obesity and exploring novel pharmacological treatments targeting the central melanocortin pathway.

Main Body:

Hinney's team provides a comprehensive review of genetic factors contributing to body weight regulation, emphasizing that over half of body weight variance is genetically determined. The study examines large epidemiological studies that identify parental obesity as a strong predictor for childhood obesity, mainly due to genetic rather than shared environmental factors. The authors also address the 'missing heritability' issue in complex diseases like obesity, where identified genetic variations explain only a small fraction of heritability. Hinney et al. highlight how genome-wide association studies have identified numerous variants associated with obesity but acknowledge that many factors remain unknown.

The research team's methods included analyzing twin and family studies, assessing polygenic risk scores, and exploring genome-wide association studies to uncover candidate genes for obesity. They also considered syndromic forms of obesity that include neurodevelopmental disorders and discussed the implications for genetic testing in clinical practice.

Conclusion:

The study by Anke Hinney's group marks significant advances in understanding the genetic underpinnings of obesity. It underscores the importance of early diagnosis and personalized treatment options for those with monogenic forms of the condition. The authors advocate for reducing stigmatization through education on the complex genetics of body weight regulation, which could ultimately help in early and correct diagnosis leading to more effective prevention and treatment approaches for childhood obesity.

Quality of Life Improvements Following One Year of Setmelanotide in Children and Adult Patients with Bardet–Biedl Syndrome: Phase 3 Trial Results [100]

This is a machine-generated summary of:

Forsythe, Elizabeth; Haws, Robert M.; Argente, Jesús; Beales, Philip; Martos-Moreno, Gabriel Á.; Dollfus, Hélène; Chirila, Costel; Gnanasakthy, Ari; Buckley, Brieana C.; Mallya, Usha G.; Clément, Karine; Haqq, Andrea M.: Quality of life improvements following one year of setmelanotide in children and adult patients with Bardet–Biedl syndrome: phase 3 trial results [100]

Published in: Orphanet Journal of Rare Diseases (2023)

Link to original: https://doi.org/10.1186/s13023-022-02602-4

If you want to cite the papers, please refer to the original.

For technical reasons we could not place the page where the original quote is coming from.

Research highlights

Background: Bardet–Biedl syndrome (BBS) is a rare genetic disorder marked by obesity, ciliary dysfunction, and multiorgan impairment. Despite its varying prevalence and autosomal recessive inheritance pattern, a molecular diagnosis confirms BBS in approximately 80% of cases. Hyperphagia and obesity are central to BBS, with most patients displaying symptoms in the first year of life, approximately 70% experience obesity or overweight by the age of 5 years, and ≥90% over the age of 6 years. Now, a new study by Elizabeth Forsythe et al. investigates the impact of the melanocortin-4 receptor agonist setmelanotide on health-related quality of life (HRQOL) in individuals with BBS.

Main Body: Forsythe and her team conducted a multicenter Phase 3 trial with a double-blind, placebo-controlled period followed by open-label treatment to assess setmelanotide's efficacy in reducing body weight and hunger scores in BBS patients. The study included participants aged ≥6 years with clinical diagnosis of BBS or Alström syndrome and obesity: patients with BMI ≥30 kg/m^2 (age ≥16 years) or weight >97th percentile (age 6 to <16 years). Patients were randomized to receive setmelanotide or placebo, with the primary endpoint being proportion of patients aged ≥ 12 years who achieved a ≥10% reduction in body weight from baseline after 52 weeks of treatment. HRQOL was measured using age-specific Pediatric Quality of Life Inventory assessments for children and adolescents, while adults used the Impact of Weight on Quality of Life Questionnaire-Lite. The researchers found that after one year of treatment, there were clinically significant reductions in body weight and hunger scores alongside improvements in HRQOL across multiple domains.

Advances/Future Directions: The study by Forsythe et al. marks a significant advance in the management of BBS-related obesity and hyperphagia. Most patients with impaired HRQOL at baseline reported meaningful improvements after 52 weeks of setmelanotide treatment. These findings not only highlight the potential for setmelanotide to improve physical function and psychosocial well-being but also underscore the importance of addressing the substantial HRQOL burden experienced by patients with BBS. As Forsythe notes, "The physical and psychosocial effects of BBS on patients and their families are complex," indicating that while setmelanotide offers promising benefits, comprehensive, multidisciplinary care strategies remain essential. Future research should continue to explore the relationship between weight management interventions and quality of life improvements to further support individuals living with this challenging condition.

Interview-Based Patient- and Caregiver-Reported Experiences of Hunger and Improved Quality of Life with Setmelanotide Treatment in Bardet-Biedl Syndrome [101]

This is a machine-generated summary of:

Ervin, Claire; Norcross, Lindsey; Mallya, Usha G.; Fehnel, Sheri; Mittleman, Robert S.; Webster, Matthew; Haqq, Andrea M.; Haws, Robert M.: Interview-Based Patient- and Caregiver-Reported Experiences of Hunger and Improved Quality of Life with Setmelanotide Treatment in Bardet-Biedl Syndrome [101]

Published in: Advances in Therapy (2023)

Link to original: https://doi.org/10.1007/s12325-023-02443-y

If you want to cite the papers, please refer to the original.

For technical reasons we could not place the page where the original quote is coming from.

Research highlights

Key Summary Points

Bardet-Biedl syndrome (BBS) is a rare genetic disorder with significant health and quality of life impacts due to symptoms like severe obesity and hyperphagia. Despite the known consequences, research on targeted treatments for these symptoms in BBS has been limited. Now a new study by Claire Ervin and colleagues explores the effects of setmelanotide, a treatment that addresses hyperphagia and obesity in BBS patients, providing insights into its impact on health-related quality of life (HRQOL) for both patients and their caregivers.

The study involved qualitative interviews with BBS patients (age atleast 16 years) or their caregivers who had participated in phase 2 or 3 clinical trials of setmelanotide. The interviews aimed to characterize the severity of hyperphagia and obesity in BBS patients and its effects on HRQOL before and during treatment. The methods were thorough, ensuring participants had firsthand experience with the drug's effects and could provide informed perspectives. The researchers used thematic analysis to identify patterns in the interview data, revealing consistent experiences among participants.

Ervin et al.'s findings highlight the profound burden that hyperphagia places on individuals with BBS and their families. The study reports that setmelanotide treatment led to significant improvements in hyperphagia symptoms, weight management, and overall HRQOL. Patients experienced enhanced control over their eating habits, reduced obsessive food-related behaviors, and weight loss. These changes also positively affected family dynamics, emotional well-being, and social interactions. The research underscores the importance of treatments like setmelanotide that can have life-changing implications for those affected by BBS. Future research may focus on long-term outcomes of hyperphagia and obesity and treatments that can impact the HRQOL in these patients.

Diagnostic and Therapeutic Odyssey of Two Patients with Compound Heterozygous Leptin Receptor Deficiency [102]

This is a machine-generated summary of:

Zorn, Stefanie; von Schnurbein, Julia; Kohlsdorf, Katja; Denzer, Christian; Wabitsch, Martin: Diagnostic and therapeutic odyssey of two patients with compound heterozygous leptin receptor deficiency [102]

Published in: Molecular and Cellular Pediatrics (2020)

Link to original: https://doi.org/10.1186/s40348-020-00107-3

If you want to cite the papers, please refer to the original.

For technical reasons we could not place the page where the original quote is coming from.

Research highlights

Obesity in children and adolescents is not only a risk factor for physical health issues but also impairs psychological and social development. While lifestyle factors contribute to obesity, severe early-onset cases are often linked to genetic variations that disrupt the leptin-melanocortin signaling pathway, crucial for regulating hunger and satiety. Despite growing knowledge about these genetic influences, there remains a gap in early identification and treatment of monogenic obesity. Now a new study by Stefanie Zorn et al. has identified compound heterozygous variants in the leptin receptor gene (LEPR) as the cause of severe early-onset obesity in two patients, providing insights into potential treatments.

Zorn's team conducted a thorough investigation into the patients' medical histories, which included persistent hyperphagia and unsuccessful weight loss attempts through various interventions, including bariatric surgery. The researchers utilized polymerase chain reaction amplification and Sanger sequencing of LEPR gene coding exons to reveal that both patients had compound heterozygous variants leading to LEPR dysfunction. This discovery confirmed the genetic basis of their condition, which had previously eluded diagnosis despite extensive testing. The study underscores the importance of considering monogenic causes in cases of extreme early-onset obesity and highlights the potential for targeted pharmacological interventions.

The findings by Zorn et al. represent a significant advance in understanding and managing monogenic obesity. The identification of LEPR gene mutations offers relief to patients and families by providing a clear diagnosis and paving the way for novel treatments like setmelanotide, an agonist affecting the leptin-melanocortin pathway currently under clinical trial. This research emphasizes the necessity for early genetic testing in children with severe obesity to avoid protracted diagnostic odysseys and ineffective treatments. Looking forward, these insights could lead to more effective management strategies for individuals with monogenic obesity, reducing the burden of this condition on patients and healthcare systems alike.

Metreleptin: First Global Approval [103]

This is a machine-generated summary of:

Chou, Ken; Perry, Caroline M.: Metreleptin: First Global Approval [103]

Published in: Drugs (2013)

Link to original: https://doi.org/10.1007/s40265-013-0074-7

If you want to cite the papers, please refer to the original.

For technical reasons we could not place the page where the original quote is coming from.

Research highlights

Lipodystrophy syndromes are a spectrum of rare disorders characterized by the abnormal distribution or lack of adipose tissue, leading to severe metabolic abnormalities or complications. Despite the classification into various types based on genetic and clinical features, effective treatments have been elusive, leaving a significant knowledge gap in managing the associated metabolic abnormalities.

Now a breakthrough has been achieved in treating these disorders with the approval of metreleptin, a recombinant analogue of human leptin, by the Japanese Ministry of Health, Labour and Welfare.

The study conducted by the Kyoto Graduate School of Medicine and supported by Shionogi focused on metreleptin as a potential therapy for lipodystrophy patients. Metreleptin works by addressing the leptin deficiency observed in these patients, thereby ameliorating their metabolic complications. The research involved an investigator-initiated trial that led to the drug's approval for subcutaneous administration in varying doses based on patient demographics. The clinical evidence suggests that metreleptin significantly improves metabolic parameters in lipodystrophy patients.

The approval of metreleptin marks a significant advance in the treatment of lipodystrophy syndromes. It offers an effective therapy option for managing associated metabolic abnormalities. Further clinical trials and regulatory efforts are expected to make metreleptin available to more patients worldwide, potentially transforming the quality of life and prognosis for those living with this challenging condition.

Metreleptin in Lipodystrophy: A Profile of Its Use [104]

This is a machine-generated summary of:

Deeks, Emma: Metreleptin in lipodystrophy: a profile of its use [104]

Published in: Drugs & Therapy Perspectives (2019)

Link to original: https://doi.org/10.1007/s40267-019-00622-y

If you want to cite the papers, please refer to the original.

For technical reasons we could not place the page where the original quote is coming from.

Research highlights

Lipodystrophies are rare disorders characterized by the loss of adipose tissue, leading to severe metabolic complications such as diabetes, hypertriglyceridemia, non-alcoholic fatty liver disease (NAFLD), non-alcoholic steatohepatitis (NASH), pancreatitis and other metabolic/endocrine abnormalities. Despite available treatments targeting individual metabolic issues, a comprehensive therapy addressing the root cause of lipodystrophy has been elusive. Now a new study by Emma Deeks delves into the efficacy and safety of metreleptin, a recombinant analogue of human leptin, as a potential game-changer in the treatment of lipodystrophy.

This study provides an in-depth analysis of metreleptin's role in managing lipodystrophy. Metreleptin works by binding to leptin receptors, mimicking the hormone's physiological effects, which include regulating appetite and improving lipid and glucose metabolism. The study employed robust methods, including integrated analyses of clinical trials and real-world data, to assess metreleptin's impact on metabolic control in patients with generalized and partial lipodystrophy. The findings are promising: significant improvements in glycemic control, hypertriglyceridemia and insulin sensitivity were observed, with some patients able to reduce or discontinue conventional diabetes and lipid-lowering medications. Moreover, metreleptin showed potential benefits for hepatic and renal outcomes, although its effects on energy expenditure remain unclear.

The study by Deek suggests a significant advance in the treatment of lipodystrophy. Metreleptin not only improves metabolic parameters but also offers potential benefits for associated liver disease and overall survival rates. Looking forward, the long-term efficacy of metreleptin, particularly concerning antibody development against the therapy, warrants further investigation. As per the study, while metreleptin is generally well tolerated with a consistent safety profile across age groups, understanding the long-term impact of immunogenicity (development of antibodies against leptin in metreleptin recipients) on its effectiveness is crucial. This research paves the way for future studies that could solidify metreleptin's role as a cornerstone therapy for lipodystrophy and improve patient outcomes significantly.

Intensive Management of Obesity in People with Prader-Willi Syndrome [105]

This is a machine-generated summary of:

Nolan, Brendan J.; Proietto, Joseph; Sumithran, Priya: Intensive management of obesity in people with Prader-Willi syndrome [105]

Published in: Endocrine (2022)

Link to original: https://doi.org/10.1007/s12020-022-03064-1

If you want to cite the papers, please refer to the original.

For technical reasons we could not place the page where the original quote is coming from.

Research highlights

Prader-Willi syndrome (PWS) is a complex genetic disorder characterized by hyperphagia, obesity, intellectual impairment, and short stature leading to significant health complications. Despite the known benefits of strict dietary control, there is a paucity of data on the efficacy and safety of intensive medical weight loss interventions in this population. Now a new study by Brendan J. Nolan and colleagues provides valuable insights into the outcomes of such interventions for individuals with PWS.

Nolan's retrospective review at Austin Health in Melbourne analyzed electronic medical records of PWS patients undergoing intensive weight loss treatments, including very-low energy diets (VLEDs) and pharmacotherapy. The study spanned January 2010 to April 2021, assessing weight outcomes and potential adverse effects. Patients were prescribed either full VLED programs or partial ones complemented by pharmacotherapy (phentermine-topiramate or Naltrexone-bupropion or liraglutide) aimed at appetite reduction. The effectiveness of these interventions was measured using statistical analyses, with significant weight loss considered a primary outcome. Despite the self-funded nature of these treatments in Australia, the study offers a real-world perspective on managing obesity in PWS.

The findings revealed that while most patients achieved significant weight loss during treatment, long-term maintenance was challenging, with only a fraction sustaining $\geq$10% weight loss at their last follow-up. Pharmacotherapies such as GLP-1 receptor agonists showed promise for tolerability. Adverse effects led to discontinuation in some cases, particularly with phentermine and topiramate. Nolan's work underscores the complexity of treating obesity in PWS and suggests that while intensive interventions can be effective, adherence remains a critical barrier to sustained success. The study advocates for further research into long-term controlled trials and newer pharmacological agents to improve outcomes for those with PWS.

Understanding the Patient Experience of Hunger and Improved Quality of Life with Setmelanotide Treatment in POMC and LEPR Deficiencies [106]

This is a machine-generated summary of:

Wabitsch, Martin; Fehnel, Sheri; Mallya, Usha G.; Sluga-O'Callaghan, Martina; Richardson, David; Price, Mark; Kühnen, Peter: Understanding the Patient Experience of Hunger and Improved Quality of Life with Setmelanotide Treatment in POMC and LEPR Deficiencies [106]

Published in: Advances in Therapy (2022)

Link to original: https://doi.org/10.1007/s12325-022-02059-8

If you want to cite the papers, please refer to the original.

For technical reasons we could not place the page where the original quote is coming from.

Research highlights

Key Summary Points

Obesity, particularly severe forms associated with genetic disorders, significantly diminishes health-related quality of life (HRQOL) and is often accompanied by psychological issues. The melanocortin receptor 4 (MC4R) pathways, which includes genes like pro-opiomelanocortin (POMC) and leptin receptor (LEPR), plays a crucial role in regulating hunger and energy balance. Mutations in this pathway can lead to insatiable hunger (hyperphagia) and severe obesity. Now a new study by Martin Wabitsch and colleagues has explored the impact of the drug setmelanotide on patients with obesity due to POMC and LEPR deficiencies, revealing not just weight loss but also improvements in HRQOL.

Wabitsch's team conducted qualitative interviews with patients who had participated in phase 3 clinical trials for setmelanotide and were part of an ongoing open-label extension. These interviews aimed to understand changes in hyperphagia and eating patterns post-treatment. The methods included detailed discussions about patients' experiences of hunger before and after treatment, their eating habits, and the psychological burden of hyperphagia. The study found that setmelanotide significantly reduced patients' hunger scores and helped maintain weight loss, leading to enhanced HRQOL.

The main advances from this research are the qualitative insights into the patient experience of hyperphagia and the subsequent improvements following setmelanotide treatment. Wabitsch et al.'s work highlights the profound personal significance of these changes for patients, who reported not only physical benefits but also emotional and social improvements.

MC4R Agonism Promotes Durable Weight Loss in Patients with Leptin Receptor Deficiency [107]

This is a machine-generated summary of:

Clément, Karine; Biebermann, Heike; Farooqi, I. Sadaf; Van der Ploeg, Lex; Wolters, Barbara; Poitou, Christine; Puder, Lia; Fiedorek, Fred; Gottesdiener, Keith; Kleinau, Gunnar; Heyder, Nicolas; Scheerer, Patrick; Blume-Peytavi, Ulrike; Jahnke, Irina; Sharma, Shubh; Mokrosinski, Jacek; Wiegand, Susanna; Müller, Anne; Weiß, Katja; Mai, Knut; Spranger, Joachim; Grüters, Annette; Blankenstein,

Oliver; Krude, Heiko; Kühnen, Peter: MC4R agonism promotes durable weight loss in patients with leptin receptor deficiency [107]

Published in: Nature Medicine (2018)

Link to original: https://doi.org/10.1038/s41591-018-0015-9

If you want to cite the papers, please refer to the original.

For technical reasons we could not place the page where the original quote is coming from.

Research highlights

Obesity is a complex condition influenced by genetic, environmental, and behavioral factors. Central to its regulation is the leptin–melanocortin pathway, which integrates signals from appetite-stimulating peptides like ghrelin, Neuropeptide Y, and Agouti-related peptide and MC4R pathway activation counteracts these orexigens.

Mutations in genes encoding components of this pathway, such as POMC and LEPR, result in severe obesity and hyperphagia. Previously, therapeutic options to regulate MC4R pathway were limited, with leptin administration being the only treatment for leptin-deficient patients. This study by Karine Clément and colleagues has made significant strides in addressing this issue.

Clément's team focused on setmelanotide, a second-generation agonist of MC4R that has shown promise in treating individuals with POMC deficiency by reducing hyperphagia and body weight without severe side effects. The researchers hypothesized that LEPR signaling deficiencies due to LEPR gene mutations causing impaired activation of POMC neurons could be similarly addressed with setmelanotide therapy. Their study involved an investigator-initiated phase 2 trial with subjects who had confirmed homozygous loss-of-function mutations in LEPR. The trial demonstrated that setmelanotide significantly reduced hunger and body weight in these individuals. The methods included careful dose escalation and monitoring. In one of the subjects, even after bariatric surgery had failed to produce lasting results, setmelanotide led to substantial weight loss and appetite control.

The main advances of this research are the demonstration of setmelanotide's efficacy in reducing hyperphagia and body weight in individuals with LEPR deficiency, extending the benefits observed in POMC deficiency cases. Clément notes that the treatment was well tolerated with only mild adverse events reported. This study not only provides hope for those with LEPR mutations but also suggests that others with monogenic obesity due to mutations in other genes (POMC) encoding MC4R pathway component mutations may benefit from setmelanotide treatment. Looking forward, Clément's team aims to understand the underlying mechanisms of setmelanotide's clinical effects better, which could improve personalized treatment regimens and aid in developing new agonists. The potential for broader application of this therapy offers an exciting prospect for addressing certain forms of genetic obesity.

Bibliography

1. Geserick M, et al. Acceleration of BMI in early childhood and risk of sustained obesity. N Engl J Med. 2018;379:1303–12. This study adresses the question of whether there is a critical age window for the manifestation of childhood obesity
2. Vogel M, et al. Age- and weight group-specific weight gain patterns in children and adolescents during the 15 years before and during the COVID-19 pandemic. Int J Obes. 2021;46:144–52.
3. Nogueira-de-Almeida CA, et al. COVID-19 and obesity in childhood and adolescence: a clinical review. J Pediatr. 2020;96:546–58.
4. The Lancet Public Health. Childhood obesity beyond COVID-19. Lancet Public Heal. 2021;6:e534. A large study analysing the obesity and COVID-19 pandemics in childhood
5. Hilbert A. Weight stigma reduction and genetic determinism. PLoS One. 2016;11:e0162993.
6. Maes HH, Neale MC, Eaves LJ. Genetic and environmental factors in relative body weight and human adiposity. Behav Genet. 1997;27:325–51.
7. Hinney A, et al. Genome wide association (GWA) study for early onset extreme obesity supports the role of fat mass and obesity associated gene (FTO) variants. PLoS One. 2007;2:e1361.
8. Khera AV, et al. Polygenic prediction of weight and obesity trajectories from birth to adulthood. Cell. 2019;177:587–596.e9.
9. Hinney A, Hebebrand J. Polygenic obesity in humans. Obes Facts. 2008;1:35–42.
10. Yengo L, et al. Meta-analysis of genome-wide association studies for height and body mass index in ~700000 individuals of European ancestry. Hum Mol Genet. 2018;27:3641–9.
11. Denzer C, et al. Pubertal development in obese children and adolescents. Int J Obes. 2007;31:1509–19.
12. de Groot CJ, et al. Determinants of advanced bone age in childhood obesity. Horm Res Paediatr. 2017;87:254–63.
13. Kohlsdorf K, et al. Early childhood BMI trajectories in monogenic obesity due to leptin, leptin receptor, and melanocortin 4 receptor deficiency. Int J Obes. 2018;42:1602–9.
14. Kleinendorst L, et al. Identifying underlying medical causes of pediatric obesity: results of a systematic diagnostic approach in a pediatric obesity center. PLoS One. 2020;15:e0244508.
15. Styne DM, et al. Pediatric obesity-assessment, treatment, and prevention: an Endocrine Society clinical practice guideline. J Clin Endocrinol Metab. 2017;102:709–57.
16. Montague CT, et al. Congenital leptin deficiency is associated with severe early-onset obesity in humans. Nature. 1997;387:903–8. The first description of leptin deficiency in humans
17. O'Rahilly S, et al. Impaired processing of prohormones associated with abnormalities of glucose homeostasis and adrenal function. N Engl J Med. 1995;333:1386–91.
18. Jackson RS, et al. Obesity and impaired prohormone processing associated with mutations in the human prohormone convertase 1 gene. Nat Genet. 1997;16:303–6.
19. Jackson RS, et al. Small-intestinal dysfunction accompanies the complex endocrinopathy of human proprotein convertase 1 deficiency. J Clin Invest. 2003;112:1550–60.
20. Farooqi IS, et al. Hyperphagia and early-onset obesity due to a novel homozygous missense mutation in prohormone convertase 1/3. J Clin Endocrinol Metab. 2007;92:3369–73.
21. Dempfle A, et al. Large quantitative effect of melanocortin-4 receptor gene mutations on body mass index. J Med Genet. 2004;41:795–800.
22. Kühnen P, et al. Proopiomelanocortin deficiency treated with a melanocortin-4 receptor agonist. N Engl J Med. 2016;375:240–6. The first report on the weight-lowering effects of the MC4R agonist setmelanotide in patients with POMC deficiency
23. Collet TH, et al. Evaluation of a melanocortin-4 receptor (MC4R) agonist (setmelanotide) in MC4R deficiency. Mol Metab. 2017;6:1321–9.
24. Markham A. Setmelanotide: first approval. Drugs. 2021;81:397–403.
25. Ryan DH. Setmelanotide: what does it mean for clinical care of patients with obesity? Lancet Diabetes Endocrinol. 2020;8:933–5.

26. Müller TD, Clemmensen C, Finan B, DiMarchi RD, Tschöp MH. Anti-obesity therapy: from rainbow pills to polyagonists. Pharmacol Rev. 2018;70:712–46.
27. Day JW, et al. A new glucagon and GLP-1 co-agonist eliminates obesity in rodents. Nat Chem Biol. 2009;5:749–57.
28. Zhu L, et al. Leptin gene-targeted editing in ob/ob mouse adipose tissue based on the CRISPR/Cas9 system. J Genet Genomics. 2021;48:134–46.
29. Shukla L, Yuan Y, Shayan R, Greening DW, Karnezis T. Fat therapeutics: the clinical capacity of adipose-derived stem cells and exosomes for human disease and tissue regeneration. Front Pharmacol. 2020;11:158.
30. Wabitsch M, Fehnel S, Mallya UG, Sluga-O'Callaghan M, Richardson D, Price M, et al. Understanding the patient experience of hunger and improved quality of life with setmelanotide treatment in POMC and LEPR deficiencies. Adv Ther. 2022;39:1–12.
31. Ervin C, Norcross L, Mallya UG, Fehnel S, Mittleman RS, Haqq AM, et al. Patient- and caregiver-reported experiences of hyperphagia in Bardet-Biedl syndrome before and during setmelanotide treatment. In: Presented at the pediatric endocrine society annual meeting; 2022. April 28–May 1; virtual
32. Haws RM, Gordon G, Han JC, Yanovski JA, Yuan G, Stewart MW. The efficacy and safety of setmelanotide in individuals with Bardet-Biedl syndrome or Alstrom syndrome: phase 3 trial design. Contemp Clin Trials Commun. 2021;22:100780.
33. Varni JW. Scaling and scoring of the Pediatric Quality of Life Inventory: PedsQL. Version 20. Mapi Research Trust https://www.pedsql.org/PedsQL-Scoring.pdf. Accessed 18 Mar 2022.
34. Kühnen P, Wabitsch M, von Schnurbein J, Chirila C, Mallya UG, Callahan P, et al. Quality of life outcomes in two phase 3 trials of setmelanotide in patients with obesity due to LEPR or POMC deficiency. Orphanet J Rare Dis. 2022;17(1):38.
35. Forsythe E, Beales PL. Bardet–Biedl syndrome. Eur J Hum Genet. 2013;21(1):8–13.
36. Geets E, Meuwissen MEC, Van Hul W. Clinical, molecular genetics and therapeutic aspects of syndromic obesity. Clin Genet. 2019;95(1):23–40.
37. Lindstrand A, Frangakis S, Carvalho CM, Richardson EB, McFadden KA, Willer JR, et al. Copy-number variation contributes to the mutational load of Bardet–Biedl syndrome. Am J Hum Genet. 2016;99(2):318–36.
38. Niederlova V, Modrak M, Tsyklauri O, Huranova M, Stepanek O. Meta-analysis of genotype-phenotype associations in Bardet-Biedl syndrome uncovers differences among causative genes. Hum Mutat. 2019;40(11):2068–87.
39. Shamseldin HE, Shaheen R, Ewida N, Bubshait DK, Alkuraya H, Almardawi E, et al. The morbid genome of ciliopathies: an update. Genet Med. 2020;22(6):1051–60.
40. Sherafat-Kazemzadeh R, Ivey L, Kahn SR, Sapp JC, Hicks MD, Kim RC, et al. Hyperphagia among patients with Bardet–Biedl syndrome. Pediatr Obes. 2013;8(5):e64–7.
41. Huvenne H, Dubern B, Clement K, Poitou C. Rare genetic forms of obesity: clinical approach and current treatments in 2016. Obes Facts. 2016;9(3):158–73.
42. Pomeroy J, Krentz AD, Richardson JG, Berg RL, VanWormer JJ, Haws RM. Bardet-Biedlsyndrome: weight patterns and genetics in a rare obesity syndrome. Pediatr Obes. 2021;16(2):e12703.
43. Hamlington B, Ivey LE, Brenna E, Biesecker LG, Biesecker BB, Sapp JC. Characterization of courtesy stigma perceived by parents of overweight children with Bardet-Biedl syndrome. PLoS One. 2015;10(10):e0140705.
44. Yazdi FT, Clee SM, Meyre D. Obesity genetics in mouse and human: back and forth, and back again. PeerJ. 2015;3:e856.
45. Davenport JR, Watts AJ, Roper VC, et al. Disruption of intraflagellar transport in adult mice leads to obesity and slow-onset cystic kidney disease. Curr Biol. 2007;17(18):1586–94.
46. Seo S, Guo DF, Bugge K, Morgan DA, Rahmouni K, Sheffield VC. Requirement of Bardet-Biedl syndrome proteins for leptin receptor signaling. Hum Mol Genet. 2009;18(7):1323–31.
47. Beales PL, Elcioglu N, Woolf AS, Parker D, Flinter FA. New criteria for improved diagnosis of Bardet-Biedl syndrome: results of a population survey. J Med Genet. 1999;36(6):437–46.

48. Dykens EM, Maxwell MA, Pantino E, Kossler R, Roof E. Assessment of hyperphagia in Prader-Willi syndrome. Obesity (Silver Spring). 2007;15(7):1816–26.
49. Heymsfield SB, Avena NM, Baier L, et al. Hyperphagia: current concepts and future directions proceedings of the 2nd international conference on hyperphagia. Obesity (Silver Spring). 2014;22(suppl 1):S1–17.
50. Forsythe E, Haws R, Argente J, et al. Quality of life in patients with Bardet-Biedl syndrome in a setmelanotide phase 3 trial. Presented at ObesityWeek; November 1–5; 2021. Virtual
51. Robert Koch-Institut. Overweight and obesity among children and adolescents in Germany. Results of the cross-sectional KiGGS Wave 2 study and trends; 2018. https://doi.org/10.17886/RKI-GBE-2018-022.
52. Siebert MF, Baumann A, Wabitsch M. Federal act on participation: opportunities for people with severe obesity. Dtsch Med Wochenschr. 2020;145:863–7. https://doi.org/10.1055/a-1146-1180.
53. Clément K, Vaisse C, Lahlou N, et al. A mutation in the human leptin receptor gene causes obesity and pituitary dysfunction. Nature. 1998;392:398–401. https://doi.org/10.1038/32911.
54. Nunziata A, Funcke J-B, Borck G, et al. Functional and phenotypic characteristics of human leptin receptor mutations. J Endoc Soc. 2019;3:27–41. https://doi.org/10.1210/js.2018-00123.
55. Clément K, Biebermann H, Farooqi IS, et al. MC4R agonism promotes durable weight loss in patients with leptin receptor deficiency. Nat Med. 2018;24:551–5. https://doi.org/10.1038/s41591-018-0015-9.
56. Kleinendorst L, Abawi O, van der Kamp HJ, et al. Leptin receptor deficiency: a systematic literature review and prevalence estimation based on population genetics. Eur J Endocrinol. 2020;182:47–56. https://doi.org/10.1530/EJE-19-0678.
57. Nizard J, Dommergues M, Clément K. Pregnancy in a woman with a leptin-receptor mutation. N Engl J Med. 2012;366:1064–5. https://doi.org/10.1056/NEJMc1200116.
58. Huvenne H, Le Beyec J, Pépin D, et al. Seven novel deleterious LEPR mutations found in early-onset obesity: a Δexon6–8 shared by subjects from Reunion Island, France, suggests a founder effect. J Clin Endocrinol Metab. 2015;100:E757–66. https://doi.org/10.1210/jc.2015-1036.
59. Le Beyec J, Cugnet-Anceau C, Pépin D, et al. Homozygous leptin receptor mutation due to uniparental disomy of chromosome 1: response to bariatric surgery. J Clin Endocrinol Metab. 2013;98:E397–402. https://doi.org/10.1210/jc.2012-2779.
60. Vos N, Oussaada SM, Cooiman MI, Kleinendorst L, Ter Horst KW, Hazebroek EJ, et al. Bariatric surgery for monogenic non-syndromic and syndromic obesity disorders. Curr Diab Rep. 2020;20(9):44.
61. Cooiman MI, Kleinendorst L, Aarts EO, et al. Genetic obesity and bariatric surgery outcome in 1014 patients with morbid obesity. Obes Surg. 2020;30:470–7. https://doi.org/10.1007/s11695-019-04184-w.
62. Farooqi IS, Jebb SA, Langmack G, et al. Effects of recombinant leptin therapy in a child with congenital leptin deficiency. N Engl J Med. 1999;341:879–84. https://doi.org/10.1056/NEJM199909163411204.
63. Brandt S, Schnurbein J, Lennerz B, et al. Methylphenidate in children with monogenic obesity due to LEPR or MC4R deficiency improves feeling of satiety and reduces BMI-SDS—a case series. Pediatr Obes. 2020;15:e12577. https://doi.org/10.1111/ijpo.12577.
64. Denzer C, Denzer F, Lennerz BS, et al. Treatment of hypothalamic obesity with dextroamphetamine: a case series. Obes Facts. 2019;12:91–102. https://doi.org/10.1159/000495851.
65. Oral EA, Chan JL. Rationale for leptin-replacement therapy for severe lipodystrophy. Endocr Pract. 2010;16(2):324–33.
66. Oral EA, Simha V, Ruiz E, et al. Leptin-replacement therapy for lipodystrophy. N Engl J Med. 2002;346:570–8.
67. Beltrand J, Beregszaszi M, Chevenne D, et al. Metabolic correction induced by leptin replacement treatment in young children with Berardinelli-Seip congenital lipoatrophy. Pediatrics. 2007;120:e291–6.

68. Amylin Pharmaceuticals Inc. Amylin completes biologics license application for metreleptin to treat diabetes and/or hypertriglyceridemia in patients with rare forms of lipodystrophy [media release]. 03 Apr 2012. http://www.amylin.com. Accessed 22 May 2013.
69. Amylin Pharmaceuticals Inc. Amylin submits clinical and nonclinical sections of rolling biologics license application for metreleptin to treat rare forms of lipodystrophy [media release]. 20 Dec 2010. http://www.amylin.com. Accessed 22 May 2013.
70. Shionogi Co Ltd. Shionogi Filed a New Drug Application for Recombinant Human Leptin for Lipodystrophy [media release]. 01 Aug 2012. http://www.shionogi.co.jp/ir_en/news/detail/e_120801.pdf. Accessed 22 May 2013.
71. Sekhar RV, Jahoor F, Iyer D, et al. Leptin replacement therapy does not improve the abnormal lipid kinetics of hypoleptinemic patients with HIV-associated lipodystrophy syndrome. Metabolism. 2012;61(10):1395–403.
72. Jazet I, Jonker J, Wijngaarden M, et al. Therapy resistant diabetes mellitus and lipodystrophy: leptin therapy leads to improvement. Ned Tijdschr Geneeskd. 2013;154(4):A5482.
73. Brown RJ, Araujo-Vilar D, Cheung PT, et al. The diagnosis and management of lipodystrophy syndromes: a multi-society practice guideline. J Clin Endocrinol Metab. 2016;101(12):4500–11.
74. Simha V. Metreleptin for metabolic disorders associated with generalized or partial lipodystrophy. Expert Rev Endocrinol Metabol. 2014;9(3):205–12.
75. King MW. Adipose tissue: not just fat. 2017. https://themedicalbiochemistrypage.org/adipose-tissue.php. Accessed 25 Feb 2019.
76. Araujo-Vilar D, Santini F. Diagnosis and treatment of lipodystrophy: a step-by-step approach. J Endocrinol Investig. 2019;42(1):61–73.
77. Meehan CA, Cochran E, Kassai A, et al. Metreleptin for injection to treat the complications of leptin deficiency in patients with congenital or acquired generalized lipodystrophy. Expert Rev Clin Pharmacol. 2016;9(1):59–68.
78. Akinci B, Meral R, Oral EA. Update on therapeutic options in lipodystrophy. Curr Diabetes Rep. 2018;18(12):139.
79. Miehle K, Stumvoll M, Fasshauer M, et al. Facial soft tissue volume decreases during metreleptin treatment in patients with partial and generalized lipodystrophy. Endocrine. 2017;58(2):262–6.
80. Muniyappa R, Abel BS, Asthana A, et al. Metreleptin therapy lowers plasma angiopoietin like protein 3 in patients with generalized lipodystrophy. J Clin Lipidol. 2017;11(2):543–50.
81. Kassai A, Muniyappa R, Levenson AE, et al. Effect of leptin administration on circulating apolipoprotein CIII levels in patients with lipodystrophy. J Clin Endocrinol Metab. 2016;101(4):1790–7.
82. Levenson AE, Haas ME, Miao J, et al. Effect of leptin replacement on PCSK9 in ob/ob mice and female lipodystrophic patients. Endocrinol. 2016;157(4):1421–9.
83. Cook K, Stears A, Araujo-Vilar D, et al. Real-world experience of generalized lipodystrophy patients enrolled in the metreleptin early access program: initial results [abstract no. PSY11 + poster]. Value Health. 2018;21 (Suppl 3):S437.
84. Ajluni N, Dar M, Xu J, et al. Efficacy and safety of metreleptin in patients with partial lipodystrophy: lessons from an expanded access program. J Diabetes Metab. 2016;7(3)
85. Myalepta. (metreleptin) 3, 5.8 and 11.3 mg powder for solution for injection: EU summary of product characteristics. Windsor: Aegerion Pharmaceuticals Ltd; 2018.
86. Jensen MD, Ryan DH, Apovian CM, Ard JD, Comuzzie AG, Donato KA, Hu FB, Hubbard VS, Jakicic JM, Kushner RF, Loria CM, Millen BE, Nonas CA, Pi-Sunyer FX, Stevens J, Stevens VJ, Wadden TA, Wolfe BM, Yanovski SZ, Jordan HS, Kendall KA, Lux LJ, Mentor-Marcel R, Morgan LC, Trisolini MG, Wnek J, Anderson JL, Halperin JL, Albert NM, Bozkurt B, Brindis RG, Curtis LH, DeMets D, Hochman JS, Kovacs RJ, Ohman EM, Pressler SJ, Sellke FW, Shen WK, Smith SC Jr, Tomaselli GF. 2013 AHA/ACC/TOS guideline for the management of overweight and obesity in adults: a report of the American College of Cardiology/American Heart Association Task Force on Practice Guidelines and The

Obesity Society. Circulation. 2014;129(25 Suppl 2):S102–38. https://doi.org/10.1161/01.cir.0000437739.71477.ee.

87. Sumithran P, Prendergast LA, Haywood CJ, Houlihan CA, Proietto J. Review of 3-year outcomes of a very-low-energy diet-based outpatient obesity treatment programme. Clin Obes. 2016;6(2):101–7. https://doi.org/10.1111/cob.12135.
88. Neoh SL, Sumithran P, Haywood CJ, Houlihan CA, Lee FT, Proietto J. Combination phentermine and topiramate for weight maintenance: the first Australian experience. Med J Aust. 2014;201(4):224–6. https://doi.org/10.5694/mja13.00193.
89. Felix G, Kossoff E, Barron B, Krekel C, Testa EG, Scheimann A. The modified Atkins diet in children with Prader-Willi syndrome. Orphanet J Rare Dis. 2020;15(1):135. https://doi.org/10.1186/s13023-020-01412-w.
90. Fintini D, Grugni G, Brufani C, Bocchini S, Cappa M, Crinò A. Use of GLP-1 receptor agonists in Prader-Willi syndrome: report of six cases. Diabetes Care. 2014;37(4):e76–7. https://doi.org/10.2337/dc13-2575.
91. Senda M, Ogawa S, Nako K, Okamura M, Sakamoto T, Ito S. The glucagon-like peptide-1 analog liraglutide suppresses ghrelin and controls diabetes in a patient with Prader-Willi syndrome. Endocrine. 2012;59(10):889–94. https://doi.org/10.1507/endocrj.ej12-0074.
92. Cyganek K, Koblik T, Kozek E, Wojcik M, Starzyk J, Malecki MT. Liraglutide therapy in Prader-Willi syndrome. Diabet Med. 2011;28(6):755–6. https://doi.org/10.1111/j.1464-5491.2011.03280.x.
93. Kim YM, Lee YJ, Kim SY, Cheon CK, Lim HH. Successful rapid weight reduction and the use of liraglutide for morbid obesity in adolescent Prader-Willi syndrome. Ann Pediatr Endocrinol Metab. 2020;25(1):52–6. https://doi.org/10.6065/apem.2020.25.1.52.
94. Seetho IW, Jones G, Thomson GA, Fernando DJ. Treating diabetes mellitus in Prader-Willi syndrome with Exenatide. Diabetes Res Clin Pract. 2011;92(1):e1–2. https://doi.org/10.1016/j.diabres.2010.12.009.
95. Paisey R, Bower L, Rosindale S, Lawrence C. Successful treatment of obesity and diabetes with incretin analogue over four years in an adult with Prader–Willi syndrome. Pract Diab. 2011;28(7):306–7. https://doi.org/10.1002/pdi.1621.
96. Wilding JPH, Batterham RL, Calanna S, Davies M, Van Gaal LF, Lingvay I, McGowan BM, Rosenstock J, Tran MTD, Wadden TA, Wharton S, Yokote K, Zeuthen N, Kushner RF. Once-weekly semaglutide in adults with overweight or obesity. N Engl J Med. 2021;384(11):989–1002. https://doi.org/10.1056/NEJMoa2032183.
97. Knox JRC, Fay M, McCagg A, et al. Burden of illness associated with rare genetic disorders of obesity. Glasgow: In: Paper presented at: 26th European Congress on Obesity 2019; April 28–May 1; 2019.
98. Clement K, van den Akker E, Argente J, et al. Efficacy and safety of setmelanotide, an MC4R agonist, in individuals with severe obesity due to LEPR or POMC deficiency: single-arm, open-label, multicentre, phase 3 trials. Lancet Diabetes Endocrinol. 2020;8:960–70.
99. Hinney A, Körner A, Fischer-Posovszky P. The promise of new anti-obesity therapies arising from knowledge of genetic obesity traits. Nat Rev Endocrinol. 2022;18:623–37. https://doi.org/10.1038/s41574-022-00716-0.
100. Forsythe E, Haws RM, Argente J, Beales P, Martos-Moreno GÁ, Dollfus H, Chirila C, Gnanasakthy A, Buckley BC, Mallya UG, Clément K, Haqq AM. Quality of life improvements following one year of setmelanotide in children and adult patients with Bardet–Biedl syndrome: phase 3 trial results. Orphanet J Rare Dis. 2023;18 https://doi.org/10.1186/s13023-022-02602-4.
101. Ervin C, Norcross L, Mallya UG, Fehnel S, Mittleman RS, Webster M, Haqq AM, Haws RM. Interview-based patient- and caregiver-reported experiences of hunger and improved quality of life with setmelanotide treatment in Bardet-Biedl syndrome. Adv Ther. 2023;40:2394–411. https://doi.org/10.1007/s12325-023-02443-y.

102. Zorn S, von Schnurbein J, Kohlsdorf K, Denzer C, Wabitsch M. Diagnostic and therapeutic odyssey of two patients with compound heterozygous leptin receptor deficiency. Mol Cell Pediatr. 2020;7:1–8. https://doi.org/10.1186/s40348-020-00107-3.
103. Chou K, Perry CM. Metreleptin: first global approval. Drugs. 2013;73:989–97. https://doi.org/10.1007/s40265-013-0074-7.
104. Deeks E. Metreleptin in lipodystrophy: a profile of its use. Drugs Therap Perspect. 2019;35:201–8. https://doi.org/10.1007/s40267-019-00622-y.
105. Nolan BJ, Proietto J, Sumithran P. Intensive management of obesity in people with Prader-Willi syndrome. Endocrine. 2022;77:57–62. https://doi.org/10.1007/s12020-022-03064-1.
106. Wabitsch M, Fehnel S, Mallya UG, Sluga-O'Callaghan M, Richardson D, Price M, Kühnen P. Understanding the patient experience of hunger and improved quality of life with Setmelanotide treatment in POMC and LEPR deficiencies. Adv Ther. 2022;39:1772–83. https://doi.org/10.1007/s12325-022-02059-8.
107. Clément K, Biebermann H, Farooqi IS, Van der Ploeg L, Wolters B, Poitou C, Puder L, Fiedorek F, Gottesdiener K, Kleinau G, Heyder N, Scheerer P, Blume-Peytavi U, Jahnke I, Sharma S, Mokrosinski J, Wiegand S, Müller A, Weiß K, Mai K, Spranger J, Grüters A, Blankenstein O, Krude H, Kühnen P. MC4R agonism promotes durable weight loss in patients with leptin receptor deficiency. Nat Med. 2018;24:551–5. https://doi.org/10.1038/s41591-018-0015-9.

Chapter 6
Future Perspectives in the Management of Obesity

Shilpa Chugh Garcha and Sanjay Kalra

Over the last decade, there has been an increasing interest in the management of obesity, with many newer medications being introduced and approved by various regulatory bodies. Better understanding and advancing knowledge of the gastrointestinal, endocrine, and neurological pathways involved in the pathophysiology of obesity has also opened newer avenues for the development of novel therapies in the management of obesity and associated co-morbidities.

In this chapter, studies included explore many novel molecules undergoing clinical trials and their target receptors involved in the management of obesity. Many new classes of drugs in the management of obesity have been introduced and are under investigation. The studies included explores newer molecules including oral non-peptide GLP-1R agonists, amylin analogues, GLP-1 and amylin receptor agonists, dual amylin and calcitonin receptor agonists, triple GLP-1/GIP/glucagon receptor agonist, pramlintide-metreleptin combination, and GLP-1/glucagon co-agonists, leptin analogues, methionine aminopeptidase 2 inhibitor, lipase inhibitor, triple monoamine reuptake inhibitors, fibroblast growth factor (FGF21) and neuropeptide Y antagonists. One of the studies also explored the anti-obesity vaccines.

Specifically, one of the studies highlighted the growing interest in incretin mimetics or GLP-1R agonists when used alone and or with other receptor agonists which include molecules showing synergistic effects of dual agonists that target GLP-1 and GIP receptors, and GLP-1 and glucagon receptors, and triple agonists that target GIP receptors, GLP-1R, and glucagon receptor. Incretin-mimetics have shown a significant impact in reducing body weight and have also shown positive cardiovascular outcomes.

S. C. Garcha (✉)
Sonepat, Haryana, India

S. Kalra
Department of Endocrinology, Bharti Hospital, Karnal, Haryana, India

S. C. Garcha, S. Kalra (eds.), *Drugs for Medical Management of Obesity*,
https://doi.org/10.1007/978-981-96-1651-0_6

Another study shared a comprehensive review of the efficacy of SGLT-2 inhibitors in weight loss as this group of drugs have shown a potential to cause weight loss. The study suggested that the combination of SGLT2 inhibitors with GLP 1R agonist can be a promising approach to manage weight and highlighted the importance of personalized medicine for obese individuals.

Another study explored the role of peripheral cannabinoid type-1 receptor antagonists as potential therapeutic agents in the management of obesity without causing central nervous system adverse events. As per the study, a dysregulation of the endocannabinoid system has been considered a factor in causing obesity with increased levels of endocannabinoids linked to high body mass index and metabolic disturbances.

Recently there has also been a growing interest in nutrition therapies and dietary supplements in the management of overweight and obesity. An increasing number of studies have also explored the efficacy and potential benefits of various nutrition therapies in the last few years.

In this chapter, we have also included studies exploring the beneficial effects of various nutrition therapies in weight management when taken consistently. One of the studies has explored the efficacy and safety of various dietary supplements including β-glucans, bitter orange, caffeine, calcium, capsaicin, chitosan, Coleus forskohlii, conjugated linoleic acid, fucoxanthin, garcinia cambogia, glucomannan, guargum, Hoodia gordonii, Irvingia gabonensis, Phaseolus vulgaris, and others. This study also explored the interaction between various dietary supplements and the various medications.

Another study included in this chapter explored the efficacy of whey proteins alone and when given along with high-fibre cereal products on various parameters including body composition, appetite, energy expenditure, insulin sensitivity, blood pressure and showed some interesting results.

Effects of taurine supplementation alone and along with exercise on anthropometry, body fat composition, oxidative stress markers, and inflammatory markers such as cytokines and gene expression in subcutaneous white adipose tissue in obese women have been explored by a study. Chitosan, a natural polysaccharide derived from crustacean shells has been studied in a randomized controlled trial that showed improvement in obesity parameters such as body fat, body weight and BMI and lipid and glycemic parameters and suggested as an adjunct to conventional treatments for the management of obesity.

A systemic review and meta-analysis of randomized controlled trials of dietary viscous fibers included in this chapter shared insights into the role of various types of viscous fibers in the management of obesity by lowering body weight, BMI, and body fat percentage. This study underscores the importance of various dietary fibres in the management of obesity when given along with conventional anti-obesity therapies.

There has been an interest in studying the impact of dietary fibres on nutrient status as these are known to improve satiety and hence less intake of food which can affect the levels of nutrients in the body, one of the studies included explores the impact of dietary fibres on micronutrient status over three months. Another study explores the impact of combining inulin-type fructans with physical activity to achieve improved health outcomes in individuals with obesity. Some molecules undergoing clinical trials for the management of overweight or obesity have been listed (Table 6.1).

Table 6.1 Ongoing clinical trials for newer molecules in the management of obesity

Drug/Molecule	Class of drug/Molecule	Condition	Clinical trial stage (Estimated date of completion)	Clinical Trial.gov ID
CagriSema	Cagrilintide (Amylin agonist) with Semaglutide	Obesity	Phase 3 (Oct'26) (REDEFINE 1)	NCT05567796
	Cagrilintide (Amylin agonist) with Semaglutide	Type 2 Diabetes and Excess Body Weight	Phase 3 (Jan'25) (REDEFINE 2)	NCT05394519
NNC0487-0111 (Amycretin)	GLP-1 and Amylin agonist	Obesity	Phase 1 (Dec'23)	NCT06049329
	GLP-1 and Amylin agonist	Obesity	Phase 1 (Jan'24)	NCT05369390
LY3437943 (Retatrutide)	GLP-1, GIP, and Glucagon tri agonist	Overweight or Obesity	Phase 3 (May'26) (TRIUMPH 1)	NCT05929066
HRS9531	GIP / GLP-1 Dual Agonist	Obesity	Phase 2 (Dec'25)	NCT06287437
CT-868	GIP / GLP-1 Dual Agonist	Overweight and Obese With T2DM	Phase 2 (Mar'23)	NCT05110846
Mazdutide (IBI362)	GLP-1 / Glucagon Dual agonist	Overweight or Obesity	Phase 2 (Dec'23)	NCT04904913
Bimagrumab	Monoclonal antibody directed against type II activin receptors	Overweight or Obesity	Phase 2 (Jun'25)	NCT05616013
Akkermansia Muciniphila WST01 Strain	Next-Generation Probiotics	Overweight or obese with T2DM	Phase 2 (Mar'24)	NCT04797442
Gly-200	Oral Duodenal exclusion therapy	Obesity	Phase 2 (Dec'24)	NCT06259981
RGT001-075	GLP-1 agonist	Obesity	Phase 2 (Jul'24)	NCT06277934
Survodutide	Glucagon/GLP-1 Dual Agonist	Obesity	Phase 3 (Dec'25) (SYNCHRONIZE)	NCT06176365
	Glucagon/GLP-1 Dual Agonist	Obesity	Phase 3 (Jan'26) (SYNCHRONIZE-1)	NCT06066515
	Glucagon/GLP-1 Dual Agonist	Overweight or Obese With Diabetes	Phase 3 (Jan'26) (SYNCHRONIZE-2)	NCT06066528

(continued)

Table 6.1 (continued)

Drug/Molecule	Class of drug/Molecule	Condition	Clinical trial stage (Estimated date of completion)	Clinical Trial.gov ID
Orforglipron	Non-peptide GLP 1 agonist	Obesity	Phase 3 (Jul'25) (ATTAIN-J)	NCT05931380
	Non-peptide GLP 1 agonist	Overweight or Obesity	Phase 3 (Sep'27) (ATTAIN 1)	NCT05869903
	Non-peptide GLP 1 agonist	Obesity or Overweight and Type 2 Diabetes	Phase 3 (Jun'25) (ATTAIN 2)	NCT05872620
Orforglipron (vs Insulin Glargine)	Non-peptide GLP 1 agonist	T2D and Obesity or Overweight at Increased Cardiovascular Risk	Phase 3 (Dec'25) (ACHIEVE-4)	NCT05803421
Dapiglutide	Dual GLP-1R/GLP-2R agonist	Obesity	Phase 2 (Aug'24) (DREAM)	NCT05788601
TG103	GLP-1/Fc fusion protein	Overweight or Obesity	Phase 2 (Mar'25)	NCT06226090
Tirzepatide	GIP / GLP-1 Dual Agonist	Overweight or Obesity	Phase 3 (Oct'27) (SURMOUNT-MMO)	NCT05556512
Family Based Behavioral Treatment/ Exenatide	GLP-1 agonist	Childhood Obesity	Phase 3 (May'25) BASIC 2	NCT04520490
Tocotrienols	Vitamin E	Obesity of Postmenopausal Women	Phase 1/2 (Aug'25) (VitE-obesity)	NCT03705845
INV-202	CB1R inverse agonist	Obesity and Metabolic Syndrome	Phase 2 (Mar'25)	NCT05891834
AMG 133 (maridebart cafraglutide)	GIPR antagonist conjugated to GLP-1 analogue	Overweight or Obese with or without T2DM	Phase 2 (Jan'26)	NCT05669599
Ecnoglutide (XW003)	GLP-1 agonist	Overweight or Obesity	Phase 3 (Jan'25) (SLIMMER)	NCT05813795
VK2735	Dual GLP-1/GIP R Agonist	Weight Loss	Phase 2 (Jun'24) (VENTURE)	NCT06068946
Cannabidivarin (CBDV)	Desensitize TRPV1, TRPV2 and TRPA1 channels	Prader-Willi Syndrome (PWS)	Phase 2 (Oct'24)	NCT03848481

6.1 Machine Generated Summaries

Disclaimer: The summaries in this chapter were generated from Springer Nature publications using abstractive AI auto-summarization: An abstraction-based summarizer creates new text based on deep learning. New phrases are created to summarize the content. As the constituted sentences are machine selected, they may not fully reflect the body of the work, so we strongly advise that the original content is read and cited. The auto-generated summaries were curated by the editor to meet Springer Nature publication standards.

Machine generated keywords: dietary, fiber, supplement, dietary fiber, nutritional, exercise

What Is the Pipeline for Future Medications for Obesity? [241]

This is a machine-generated summary of:

Melson E, Ashraf U, Papamargaritis D, Davies MJ. What is the pipeline for future medications for obesity? [241]

Published in: International Journal of Obesity (2024)

Link to original: https://doi.org/10.1038/s41366-024-01473-y

If you want to cite the papers, please refer to the original.

For technical reasons we could not place the page where the original quote is coming from.

Research highlights

Introduction:

Obesity, a global health crisis, affects millions and predisposes individuals to a spectrum of metabolic and mechanical complications. Despite lifestyle interventions being pivotal in obesity management, their long-term efficacy is limited, with significant weight regain common over time. Now a new study by Eka Melson and colleagues delves into the burgeoning field of obesity pharmacotherapies, focusing on entero-pancreatic hormone-based treatments. Their comprehensive review evaluates the safety and efficacy of these emerging therapies in clinical trials, offering insights into their potential to revolutionize obesity management.

Main Body:

Melson et al.'s review meticulously examines the current landscape of obesity pharmacotherapies, particularly those harnessing the regulatory functions of entero-pancreatic hormones on appetite and metabolism. The authors highlight the promising results of tirzepatide, an FDA-approved dual GLP-1 and GIP receptor agonist from the SURPASS (for diabetes) and SURMOUNT (for obesity) programme, which has shown significant weight loss outcomes in patients with and without diabetes. They also discuss various molecules based on entero-pancreatic hormones such as oral GLP-1 receptor agonists like semaglutide and novel oral non-peptide GLP-1RA such as orforglipron and danuglipron that offer alternative administration routes to injections, potentially improving patient adherence. Other novel molecules explored in the review included amylin analogues (pramlintide and cagrilintide), cagrisema (GLP-1 and amylin receptor agonist), amycretin (GLP-1 and amylin receptor agonist), triple agonist retatrutide (GLP-1/GIP/glucagon receptor agonist), GLP-1/glucagon co-agonists (mazdutide, pemvidutide, efinopegdutide, and survodutide), PYY agonists. The review methodically dissects data from early to late-phase trials, scrutinizing the impact of these therapies not only on weight loss but also on other obesity-related complications like glycaemia control in diabetes and liver fat content in steatohepatitis.

Conclusion:

The main advances underscored by Melson et al. include the marked weight loss achieved with tirzepatide and other entero-pancreatic hormone-based pharmacotherapies that approach the efficacy of bariatric surgery without its associated risks or scalability issues. Looking forward, they suggest that oral formulations could enhance convenience and adherence, broadening treatment options for patients. As per the authors, the new era in obesity pharmacotherapy will bring both clinical implications and challenges and while these therapies are transformative, their integration into clinical practice must be navigated carefully. Future research should aim to elucidate long-term effects, optimize treatment regimens, and ensure equitable access to these promising interventions.

Future Pharmacotherapy for Obesity: New Anti-obesity Drugs on the Horizon [242]

This is a machine-generated summary of:

Srivastava G, Apovian C. Future pharmacotherapy for obesity: new anti-obesity drugs on the horizon [242]

Published in: Current Obesity Reports (2018)

Link to original: https://doi.org/10.1007/s13679-018-0300-4

If you want to cite the papers, please refer to the original.

For technical reasons we could not place the page where the original quote is coming from.

Research highlights

Obesity is a critical health issue that exacerbates numerous medical conditions, leading to increased morbidity and mortality. Patients with a high body mass index (BMI) who do not respond to lifestyle interventions are often recommended for pharmacotherapy. However, the response to FDA-approved anti-obesity drugs is highly variable, and adverse effects can necessitate discontinuation of treatment. Now, a new study by Gitanjali Srivastava and Caroline Apovian addresses this challenge by reviewing emerging pharmacotherapeutics for obesity, focusing on their mechanisms of action, safety profiles, and potential clinical utility.

The author delves into the complex regulation of energy homeostasis and how an imbalance can lead to obesity. They explore the role of neurons in the hypothalamus that respond to neurohormonal signals affecting appetite and energy expenditure. The study meticulously examines various novel agents such as Setmelanotide, a melanocortin receptor agonist; velneperit, a neuropeptide Y antagonist; combination drugs like zonisamide-bupropion, cannabinoid type-1 receptor blockers, semaglutide, amylin mimetics, dual amylin and calcitonin receptor agonists [DACRA], glucose-dependent insulinotropic polypeptide (GIP) analogue, dual action GLP-1/glucagon receptor agonists, GC-Co-agonist and glucagon-GIP-GLP-1 triple agonist, peptide YY (PYY), leptin analogues (metreleptin), pramlintide-metreleptin combination, beloranib (methionine aminopeptidase 2 inhibitor), cetilistat (lipase inhibitor), triple monoamine reuptake inhibitors (tesofensine), fibroblast growth factor 21, and anti-obesity vaccines (ghrelin, somatostatin, Ad36). The methods include randomized controlled trials and in-depth analyses of drug effects on various parameters such as resting energy expenditure, food intake, and weight loss outcomes.

The research highlights significant advances in obesity pharmacotherapy. Setmelanotide shows promise for rare genetic disorders of obesity without adverse effects on heart rate or blood pressure. Velneperit's proof-of-concept suggests future potential for neuropeptide Y antagonists. The zonisamide-bupropion combination demonstrates superior efficacy compared to monotherapy with tolerable side effects. Looking forward, Srivastava et al. suggest that these novel treatments could revolutionize the management of obesity by offering targeted therapies that mitigate the limitations of current drugs. The study underscores the importance of continued research into the safety and efficacy of these agents to provide more personalized and effective treatment options for individuals struggling with obesity.

Dual and Triple Incretin-Based Co-agonists: Novel Therapeutics for Obesity and Diabetes [243]

This is a machine-generated summary of:

Gutgesell RM, Nogueiras R, Tschöp MH, Müller TD. Dual and triple incretin-based co-agonists: novel therapeutics for obesity and diabetes [243]

Published in: Diabetes Therapy (2024)

Link to original: https://doi.org/10.1007/s13300-024-01566-x

If you want to cite the papers, please refer to the original.

For technical reasons we could not place the page where the original quote is coming from.

Research highlights

Key Summary Points

The escalating global obesity and diabetes epidemic poses a significant health challenge, with obesity-related complications such as chronic kidney disease, heart disease, and liver disease reducing both the quality and quantity of life. Despite various pharmacological strategies to combat obesity, many have been limited by adverse effects or insufficient efficacy. Now a new study by Robert M. Gutgesell and colleagues explores the neuroendocrine pathways involved in body weight regulation, focusing on the potential of incretin hormones like glucagon-like peptide-1 (GLP-1) and glucose-dependent insulinotropic polypeptide (GIP) as targets for effective anti-obesity pharmacotherapies.

Introduction

Obesity and diabetes are major contributors to global morbidity and mortality, with a projected increase in diabetes prevalence by 46% by 2045. The ineffectiveness of lifestyle modifications for long-term weight management underscores the need for research into safe and effective anti-obesity drugs. Previous attempts have been hampered by side effects or limited success, highlighting the importance of understanding neuroendocrine pathways like those involving leptin and ghrelin. Gutgesell et al.'s study delves into incretin hormones, particularly GLP-1 and GIP, which have shown promise in reducing body weight and improving glucose metabolism.

Main Body

Gutgesell's team synthesized a narrative around the discovery of incretin hormones and their role in weight regulation. They detailed how GLP-1, secreted in response to food intake, not only enhances insulin secretion and decreases gastric emptying but also acts on the brain to reduce food intake. Similarly, GIP has been found to influence body weight through its actions on pancreatic cells and the central nervous system. The researchers highlighted the development of incretin agonists like exenatide, liraglutide, and semaglutide, which have transformed obesity treatment with significant reductions in body weight and improved cardiovascular outcomes.

The study also examined the potential of combining incretin hormone actions through dual agonists targeting both GLP-1 and GIP receptors, such as tirzepatide or GLP-1 and glucagon receptors. These dual agonists have demonstrated greater efficacy than single-receptor agonists in preclinical models and human trials. Furthermore, Gutgesell's team explored triagonists that simultaneously target GIPR, GLP-1R, and glucagon receptor (GCGR), showing even more promising results in reducing body weight and improving metabolic health, paving way for development of newer molecules such as HM15211 and retatrutide.

Conclusion

This review by Gutgesell et al. represent a significant step forward in obesity pharmacotherapy. By leveraging the synergistic effects of incretin hormones through dual and triagonist drugs, they offer improved efficacy compared to previous treatments. The study points towards future directions for research into the mechanisms driving weight loss with these therapies while considering long-term patient health implications. The findings suggest that we are moving closer to bridging the gap between pharmacotherapies and surgical methods for treating obesity and diabetes.

Emerging Role of SGLT-2 Inhibitors for the Treatment of Obesity [244]

This is a machine-generated summary of:

Pereira MJ, Eriksson JW. Emerging role of SGLT-2 inhibitors for the treatment of obesity [244]

Published in: Drugs (2019)

Link to original: https://doi.org/10.1007/s40265-019-1057-0

If you want to cite the papers, please refer to the original.

For technical reasons we could not place the page where the original quote is coming from.

Research highlights

Introduction:

Obesity has become a critical global health crisis, with its prevalence doubling in recent years, leading to a myriad of health complications and increased healthcare costs. Despite various treatments, including bariatric surgery and lifestyle changes, the need for more effective weight-loss therapies persists. Now a new study by Maria J. Pereira and Jan W. Eriksson delves into the potential of sodium-glucose co-transporter 2 (SGLT2) inhibitors as a treatment for obesity, both alone and in combination with other pharmacotherapies.

Main Body:

This study provides a comprehensive review of SGLT2 inhibitors' clinical effects on patients with type 2 diabetes (T2D) and obese individuals without diabetes. The study meticulously examines the efficacy of these inhibitors in promoting weight loss and improving cardiometabolic health. SGLT2 inhibitors can cause weight loss due to their ability to induce glucosuria and subsequent caloric loss. However, the study acknowledges an adaptive increase in energy intake that may counteract the weight loss benefits. Pereira's team noted that combination therapies often yield better results than monotherapy due to synergistic effects on different physiological pathways.

Conclusion:

The study by Pereira and Eriksson marks a significant advance in understanding how SGLT2 inhibitors can be optimized for treating obesity. The future of obesity treatment may well lie in personalized medicine, suggests the authors, indicating that identifying patient characteristics responsive to these therapies could enhance their effectiveness. While SGLT2 inhibitor monotherapy offers modest weight loss, its combination with appetite-reducing drugs such as GLP 1RA presents a promising strategy for substantial weight reduction. Future trials should aim at refining dose optimization, safety profiles, and lifestyle interventions to maximize therapeutic outcomes for obese patients with or without T2D.

Anti-obesity Therapy with Peripheral CB1 Blockers: From Promise to Safe(?) Practice [245]

This is a machine-generated summary of:

Quarta C, Cota D. Anti-obesity therapy with peripheral CB1 blockers: from promise to safe(?) practice [245]

Published in: International Journal of Obesity (2020)

Link to original: https://doi.org/10.1038/s41366-020-0577-8

If you want to cite the papers, please refer to the original.

For technical reasons we could not place the page where the original quote is coming from.

Research highlights

Introduction:

Evolution has fine-tuned human metabolism to store energy efficiently, a survival trait for periods of famine, that becomes maladaptive in today's world of caloric abundance and sedentary lifestyles. This mismatch contributes to the obesity epidemic, yet the biological underpinnings of energy storage and obesity remain elusive, hence, few effective long-term weight loss pharmacological interventions are available. Now a new study by Carmelo Quarta and Daniela Cota delves into the role of the endocannabinoid system (ECS) in obesity, revealing insights into peripheral cannabinoid type-1 receptor (CB1R) antagonists as potential therapeutic agents.

Main Body:

Quarta and Daniela's research builds on the understanding that ECS dysregulation is linked to obesity, with elevated endocannabinoid levels correlating with increased body mass index and metabolic disturbances such as insulin resistance and dyslipidemia. The study meticulously dissects the mechanisms by which peripheral CB1R antagonists can mitigate obesity without the neuropsychiatric side effects associated with earlier generations of ECS-targeting drugs. Considering the genetic models, pharmacological interventions, and metabolic assays, the study suggests that these peripheral blockers not only reduce body weight but also improve insulin resistance, dyslipidemia, and hepatic steatosis. The therapeutic efficacy of peripherally restricted blockers is comparable to global antagonists as per the preclinical studies which underscores their potential as safer alternatives in obesity pharmacotherapy. The authors have explored the molecule JD5037, a peripheral CB1R antagonist in this study.

Conclusion:

The main advance highlighted by this study is the demonstration that peripheral CB1R antagonists can effectively address obesity and its complications without central nervous system side effects. Looking forward, the author suggests that these novel molecules may offer a multi-faceted approach to metabolic regulation. The research paves the way for clinical trials and further exploration into how these peripheral blockers can be integrated into existing treatment paradigms or even lead to new unimolecular therapies when combined with other metabolic modulators.

Nutritionist and Obesity: Brief Overview on Efficacy, Safety, and Drug Interactions of the Main Weight-Loss Dietary Supplements [246]

This is a machine-generated summary of:

Barrea L, Altieri B, Polese B, De Conno B, Muscogiuri G, Colao A, Savastano S. Nutritionist and obesity: brief overview on efficacy, safety, and drug interactions of the main weight-loss dietary supplements [246]

Published in: International Journal of Obesity Supplements (2019)

Link to original: https://doi.org/10.1038/s41367-019-0007-3

If you want to cite the papers, please refer to the original.

For technical reasons we could not place the page where the original quote is coming from.

Research highlights

Background and Knowledge Gap:

Obesity is a global health concern intricately linked to numerous non-communicable diseases, such as heart disease, stroke, and some cancer types, and significantly impacts the quality of life and increases morbidity, mortality, and healthcare costs. While diet and lifestyle changes are universally recommended for weight management, many individuals find it challenging to sustain the lifestyle changes, leading to a common relapse into obesity. This has fueled interest in dietary weight-loss supplements as an easier alternative to conventional lifestyle modifications. However, the effectiveness and safety of these supplements, particularly in relation to drug interactions, remain poorly understood.

Key Findings:

Now a new study by Luigi Barrea and colleagues addresses this knowledge gap by providing a comprehensive review of the most commonly used weight-loss dietary supplements. This review focuses on their efficacy, safety, and potential drug interactions, offering valuable insights for healthcare providers managing obese patients.

Study Story:

The authors meticulously summarize evidence-based studies on β-glucans, bitter orange, caffeine, calcium, capsaicin, carnitine, chitosan, chromium, Coleus forskohlii, conjugated linoleic acid (CLA), fucoxanthin, garcinia cambogia, glucomannan, guar gum, Hoodia gordonii, Irvingia gabonensis (African mango), Phaseolus vulgaris, pyruvate, and raspberry ketone. They explore each supplement's efficacy in weight management and potential safety concerns. For instance, there is inconclusive data for β-glucans on satiety and weight loss and these have been shown to interact with many prescription medications. Bitter orange contains p-synephrine with cardiovascular risks similar to ephedrine. Caffeine's role in weight maintenance is supported by observational studies but lacks clinical trial confirmation and some studies have reported interaction of caffeine with other medications.

Advances and Future Directions:

The review by Barrea et al. represents a significant advance in understanding the complex interplay between dietary supplements and various medications. It underscores the need for robust clinical trials to establish clear efficacy and safety profiles for these supplements. As noted by the authors, "Many bioactive constituents remain unknown, uncharacterized, or not adequately tested in combination with one another, possibly shifting their risk-benefits balance against their use." The study advocates for informed discussions between healthcare providers and patients regarding supplement use as part of a comprehensive weight-loss strategy that prioritizes lifestyle changes over supplementation.

Effects of Whey Protein and Dietary Fiber Intake on Insulin Sensitivity, Body Composition, Energy Expenditure, Blood Pressure, and Appetite in Subjects with Abdominal Obesity [247]

This is a machine-generated summary of:

Fuglsang-Nielsen R, Rakvaag E, Langdahl B, Knudsen KE, Hartmann B, Holst JJ, Hermansen K, Gregersen S. Effects of whey protein and dietary fiber intake on insulin sensitivity, body composition, energy expenditure, blood pressure, and appetite in subjects with abdominal obesity [247]

Published in: European Journal of Clinical Nutrition (2020)
Link to original: https://doi.org/10.1038/s41430-020-00759-4

If you want to cite the papers, please refer to the original.

For technical reasons we could not place the page where the original quote is coming from.

Research highlights

Introduction:

The consumption of dairy products and cereal fiber has been inversely associated with abdominal obesity, with whey protein (WP) and dietary fiber receiving particular attention for their potential metabolic health benefits. While WP and dietary fibre has been linked to improved body composition, blood pressure, insulin resistance, and increased satiety, the long-term effects on appetite and metabolic syndrome features remain less understood. Now a new study by Rasmus Fuglsang-Nielsen et al. aims to shed light on the separate and combined effects of WP and high-fiber cereal products on insulin sensitivity, body composition, blood pressure, appetite, and energy expenditure over a 12-week period.

Main Body:

Fuglsang-Nielsen's team conducted a randomized, controlled, double-blind study as part of the MERITS project. Seventy-three participants with abdominal obesity were recruited and divided into groups receiving either WP plus high fiber, WP plus low fiber or maltodextrin plus high fiber, maltodextrin plus low fiber.

The study maintained an energy-balanced design to focus on the metabolic effects of protein and fiber intake without weight change interference. "We hypothesized that the combination of high-protein and high-fiber diets would have additive beneficial effects on these outcomes," explains Fuglsang-Nielsen.

The participants' adherence to the diet was closely monitored through self-reported journals, dietary records, and biochemical markers. Despite rigorous methodology, the study found no significant impact on insulin sensitivity, blood pressure, energy expenditure, incretins, or body composition from either intervention. However, an interesting outcome was observed in appetite modulation; WP supplementation reduced subjective hunger ratings during a high-fat meal test compared to maltodextrin.

Conclusion:

The research by Fuglsang-Nielsen et al. contributes to our understanding of dietary interventions in metabolic health by demonstrating that while WP may influence appetite sensations, it does not significantly affect insulin sensitivity, blood pressure, or body composition when combined with high-fiber cereal products in individuals with abdominal obesity over 12 weeks. The author suggests that while whey protein may help reduce hunger, its long-term benefits on this feature requires further investigation.

Taurine Supplementation in Conjunction with Exercise Modulated Cytokines and Improved Subcutaneous White Adipose Tissue Plasticity in Obese Women [248]

This is a machine-generated summary of:

De Carvalho FG, Brandao CF, Muñoz VR, Batitucci G, Tavares ME, Teixeira GR, Pauli JR, De Moura LP, Ropelle ER, Cintra DE, da Silva AS. Taurine supplementation in conjunction with exercise modulated cytokines and improved subcutaneous white adipose tissue plasticity in obese women [248]

Published in: Amino Acids (2021)

Link to original: https://doi.org/10.1007/s00726-021-03041-4

If you want to cite the papers, please refer to the original.

For technical reasons we could not place the page where the original quote is coming from.

Research highlights

Background and Key Findings:

Obesity is a complex condition that promotes adipose tissue remodeling, leading to a proinflammatory state and metabolic diseases. The low-grade chronic inflammation associated with obesity involves increased mast cells and adipose remodeling causing dysregulated adipokine secretion, impacting systemic health and causing metabolic diseases. Interventions like exercise and dietary components such as taurine—a sulfated amino acid—have been proposed as strategies to manage obesity. Now a new study by Flavia Giolo De Carvalho et al. examines the synergistic effects of taurine supplementation and exercise on oxidative stress and inflammatory markers and gene expression in subcutaneous white adipose tissue (scWAT) of obese women, revealing the benefits for obesity treatment.

Study Narrative:

The research conducted by De Carvalho's team involved obese women who were administered either taurine supplements or taurine supplements along with an exercise regimen. The study meticulously measured changes in plasma cytokine levels, oxidative stress markers, and gene expression related to taurine biosynthesis enzymes in scWAT. Taurine supplementation alone reduced plasma interleukin-6 (IL-6) levels, while its combination with exercise increased anti-inflammatory cytokines IL-10 and IL-15. Moreover, the exercise group showed reduced expression of the interleukin-1β gene in scWAT. These findings were complemented by histological analyses indicating reduced adipocyte size and increased connective tissue in scWAT post-intervention.

Advances and Future Directions:

The main advances highlighted by this study include the demonstration that taurine supplementation, particularly when combined with exercise, can positively modulate anti-inflammatory markers in plasma and scWAT along with improvement in scWAT plasticity in obese women. This intervention also led to significant remodeling of adipose tissue, suggesting a potential role for taurine in improving metabolic health through adipose tissue plasticity. De Carvalho et al.'s work opens avenues for future research to explore optimal dosing strategies and further elucidate the mechanisms by which taurine affects inflammation and metabolic regulation in human adipose tissue. The authors suggest that these findings could pave the way for new therapeutic approaches to treat obesity and prevent related metabolic disorders.

The Effects of Chitosan Supplementation on Anthropometric Indicators of Obesity, Lipid and Glycemic Profiles, and Appetite-Regulated Hormones in Adolescents with Overweight or Obesity: A Randomized, Double-Blind Clinical Trial [249]

This is a machine-generated summary of:

Fatahi S, Sayyari AA, Salehi M, Safa M, Sohouli M, Shidfar F, Santos HO. The effects of chitosan supplementation on anthropometric indicators of obesity, lipid and glycemic profiles, and appetite-regulated hormones in adolescents with overweight or obesity: a randomized, double-blind clinical trial [249]

Published in: BMC Pediatrics (2022)

Link to original: https://doi.org/10.1186/s12887-022-03590-x

If you want to cite the papers, please refer to the original.

For technical reasons we could not place the page where the original quote is coming from.

Research highlights

Introduction:

The global rise in adolescent obesity is a pressing health concern, with childhood obesity closely linked to adult obesity and associated noncommunicable diseases.

Lifestyle changes and medications are traditional interventions, however, nutrition-based therapies have adherence challenges and potential nutrient deficits call for alternative strategies. Now a new study by Somaye Fatahi and colleagues addresses this issue by exploring the impact of chitosan supplementation on appetite hormones, obesity markers, and metabolic (lipid and glycemic) profiles in overweight or obese adolescents.

Main Body:

Fatahi et al.'s double-blind randomized clinical trial, conducted at Mofid Children's Hospital in Tehran, Iran, rigorously tested the effects of chitosan—a polysaccharide derived from crustacean shells—on various health parameters. The study spanned over 12 weeks and involved adolescents who met specific inclusion criteria. Participants were randomly assigned to receive either chitosan or a placebo while adhering to dietary recommendations aimed at gradual weight loss. The researchers ensured the integrity of the trial through meticulous methods such as stratified randomization and blinding of both participants and investigators.

The intervention group received 3.0 g of chitosan powder daily (1.5 g twice daily) 30 minutes to 1 hour before meals, chosen based on previous studies and recognized as safe by the FDA. The team monitored adherence through package returns and assessed changes in anthropometric measurements, physical activity levels, dietary intake, and biochemical markers (lipid and glycemic profiles) using standardized tools and procedures.

Conclusion:

The study's findings are significant: chitosan supplementation led to notable improvements in weight management, glycemic control, lipid profiles, and appetite-regulating hormones among adolescents with overweight or obesity. These results suggest that chitosan could be a valuable adjunct to conventional treatments for adolescent obesity. However, Fatahi et al. caution that chitosan should not be seen as a standalone solution but rather as part of a comprehensive approach that includes diet and exercise under professional guidance.

Effect of Viscous Fiber Supplementation on Obesity Indicators in Individuals Consuming Calorie-Restricted Diets: A Systematic Review and Meta-analysis of Randomized Controlled Trials [250]

This is a machine-generated summary of:

Jovanovski E, Mazhar N, Komishon A, Khayyat R, Li D, Blanco Mejia S, Khan T, Jenkins AL, Smircic-Duvnjak L, Sievenpiper JL, Vuksan V. Effect of viscous fiber supplementation on obesity indicators in individuals consuming calorie-restricted diets: a systematic review and meta-analysis of randomized controlled trials [250]

Published in: European Journal of Nutrition (2020)

Link to original: https://doi.org/10.1007/s00394-020-02224-1

If you want to cite the papers, please refer to the original.

For technical reasons we could not place the page where the original quote is coming from.

Research highlights

Introduction:

Modern obesity management strategies emphasize dietary modifications to promote weight loss. Even the modest reductions in body weight significantly improving health outcomes. Dietary fiber, particularly viscous types, has been identified as a potential aid in weight control due to its effects on appetite and nutrient kinetics. Despite the known benefits, most individuals do not meet the recommended daily intake of fiber, and the impact of viscous fiber supplementation in a calorie-deficit diet remains unclear. Now a new study by Elena Jovanovski and colleagues addresses this gap by evaluating the effects of viscous fiber supplementation on body weight and other anthropometric measures within a calorie-restricted diet.

Methods:

Jovanovski et al.'s research adhered to rigorous systematic review protocols, including registration and adherence to Preferred Reporting Items for Systematic Reviews and Meta-Analysis (PRISMA) guidelines. The team conducted comprehensive searches across multiple databases, selecting randomized controlled trials (RCTs) that compared viscous fiber supplementation (agar, alginate, beta glucan, guar gum, konjac, psyllium, xanthan, or viscous fiber blend (konjac, alginate and xanthan) with non-fiber controls in calorie-deficit diets.

They meticulously extracted data, assessed study quality using the Cochrane Risk of Bias Tool, and synthesized results using meta-analytical techniques. The Grading of Recommendations Assessment, Development and Evaluation (GRADE) approach was employed to evaluate evidence certainty.

Results and Discussion:

The study's findings indicate that viscous fiber supplementation can lead to significant reductions in body weight, BMI, and body fat percentage when part of a calorie-deficit diet. Notably, the type of fiber appears to influence outcomes, with more viscous fibers showing greater efficacy. These results suggest that viscous fibers may offer a slight but clinically meaningful advantage in weight management strategies. Jovanovski et al.'s work contributes valuable insights into the role of viscous dietary fibers in obesity management and highlights the potential for simple dietary interventions to complement more weight loss regimens.

Conclusion:

Elena Jovanovski's team has provided moderate-quality evidence that viscous fiber supplementation can modestly improve weight management outcomes as an adjunct to calorie-restricted diets in adults at risk for cardiovascular disease (CVD). This research underscores the practical utility of gel-forming fibers in weight loss programs and their additional benefits for cardiometabolic health. Future research should focus on long-term trials to refine these findings and inform dietary guidelines aimed at reducing obesity-related CVD risks.

Micronutrient Status of Individuals with Overweight and Obesity Following 3 months' Supplementation with PolyGlycopleX (PGX®) or Psyllium: A Randomized Controlled Trial [251]

This is a machine-generated summary of:

Pal S, McKay J, Ho S, Jane M, Gahler RJ, Wood S. Micronutrient status of individuals with overweight and obesity following 3 months' supplementation with PolyGlycopleX (PGX®) or psyllium: a randomized controlled trial [251]

Published in: BMC Nutrition (2022)

Link to original: https://doi.org/10.1186/s40795-022-00534-7

If you want to cite the papers, please refer to the original.

For technical reasons we could not place the page where the original quote is coming from.

Research highlights

Obesity, a complex interplay of genetic and environmental factors, is exacerbated by the consumption of processed, nutrient-poor foods, leading to excess weight gain and potential micronutrient deficiencies. These deficiencies are further complicated in overweight individuals due to altered nutrient bioavailability and utilization. Now a new study by Sebely Pal and colleagues addresses the knowledge gap regarding the impact of high dietary fiber supplementation on micronutrient status in overweight and obese adults.

The research conducted at Curtin University involved overweight and obese participants who were randomized into three groups: a control group, a psyllium fiber supplement group, and a PolyGlycopleX (PGX®) fiber supplement group. Over three months, participants consumed 5 g of their assigned supplement before meals three times a day (total 15 g) without altering their usual diet. Blood samples were collected at baseline and after the intervention to assess serum micronutrient levels, while 3-day food diaries tracked dietary intake. The study's rigorous design ensured blinding of both participants and researchers to the type of supplement consumed, with adherence monitored through supplement sachet returns.

The study's findings indicate no significant differences in serum micronutrient levels between the fiber supplement groups and the control group after three months. However, within-group increases in certain micronutrients like folate suggest potential benefits from fiber supplementation. Self-reported dietary data revealed a decrease in overall nutrient intake, possibly due to the satiating effects of fiber leading to reduced food consumption. These results suggest that short-term high-fiber supplementation may not adversely affect micronutrient status in overweight individuals.

Sebely Pal's team highlights that while fiber supplements like PGX® and psyllium do not significantly alter serum micronutrient levels over three months, they may influence dietary intake patterns due to increased satiety. The research underscores the importance of considering long-term effects and varying dosages in future studies to fully understand the implications of fiber supplementation on nutrient status in weight management. As obesity continues to be a global health challenge, this study contributes valuable insights into safe weight management strategies that do not compromise micronutrient sufficiency.

Physical Activity Enhances the Improvement of Body Mass Index and Metabolism by Inulin: A Multicenter Randomized Placebo-Controlled Trial Performed in Obese Individuals [252]

This is a machine-generated summary of:

Rodriguez J, Neyrinck AM, Van Kerckhoven M, Gianfrancesco MA, Renguet E, Bertrand L, Cani PD, Lanthier N, Cnop M, Paquot N, Thissen JP, Bindels LB, Delzenne NM. Physical activity enhances the improvement of body mass index and metabolism by inulin: a multicenter randomized placebo-controlled trial performed in obese individuals [252]

Published in: BMC Medicine (2022)

Link to original: https://doi.org/10.1186/s12916-022-02299-z

If you want to cite the papers, please refer to the original.

For technical reasons we could not place the page where the original quote is coming from.

Research highlights

Background:

The burgeoning interest in prebiotics for managing obesity and metabolic disorders is underscored by studies demonstrating the benefits of prebiotics like Inulin-type fructans (ITF) on various health parameters. While ITF intake has been linked to improved gut barrier function, glucose intolerance, postprandial hypertriglyceridemia, endothelial dysfunction, and hepatic steatosis in rodent obesity models, human intervention studies also support ITF's role in managing metabolic disorders. However, the variability in metabolic response to dietary interventions raises questions about the influence of individual factors such as gut microbiota composition, dietary fiber intake, and medications like metformin. Now a new study by Julie Rodriguez and colleagues addresses the interplay between physical activity (PA) and prebiotic efficacy, hypothesizing that PA could modulate both gut microbiota and the effectiveness of prebiotics in obese individuals.

Main Text:

Rodriguez et al. embarked on a comprehensive investigation combining preclinical and clinical approaches to unravel the interaction between inulin intake and PA within the context of obesity. Their methodology involved a multicentric, single-blind placebo-controlled trial with obese patients undergoing inulin supplementation alongside dietary advice to consume fructan-rich vegetables. The study was meticulously designed with stringent inclusion criteria and robust randomization protocols, ensuring reliable data collection for gut microbiota composition and various metabolic parameters. Simultaneously, an intervention study with high-fat diet-fed mice examined molecular mechanisms behind the metabolic and microbial outcomes of combined PA and inulin intervention. The researchers' findings were striking: increased PA during prebiotic supplementation significantly enhanced weight loss and metabolic parameters while improving gastrointestinal tolerance.

Conclusion:

The study by Rodriguez et al. marks a significant advance in understanding how physical activity can amplify the health benefits of prebiotic based nutritional interventions. Their work suggests that incorporating voluntary PA can maximize clinical outcomes from prebiotic interventions like ITF supplementation, particularly concerning body weight management and glucose homeostasis and its effect on total cholesterol and liver enzymes. Looking forward, these insights pave the way for future research to explore specific exercise programs that could further optimize prebiotic efficacy in obesity management. The authors underscored the potential of combining dietary strategies with physical activity to achieve better health outcomes in obese individuals.

Bibliography

1. Bergmann NC, Davies MJ, Lingvay I, Knop FK. Semaglutide for the treatment of overweight and obesity: a review. Diabetes Obes Metab. 2023;25:18–35.
2. Melson E, Alexander A, Miras D, Papamargaritis D. Future therapies for obesity. Clin Med. 2023;23:337–46.
3. Thethi TK, Pratley R, Meier JJ. Efficacy, safety and cardiovascular outcomes of once-daily oral semaglutide in patients with type 2 diabetes: the PIONEER programme. Diabetes Obes Metab. 2020;22:1263–77.
4. Pfizer announces topline phase 2b results of oral GLP-1R agonist, danuglipron, in adults with obesity | Pfizer. 2023. https://www.pfizer.com/news/press-release/press-release-detail/pfizer-announces-topline-phase-2b-results-oral-glp-1r
5. Knop FK, Aroda VR, do Vale RD, Holst-Hansen T, Laursen PN, Rosenstock J, et al. Oral semaglutide 50 mg taken once per day in adults with overweight or obesity (OASIS 1): a randomised, double-blind, placebo-controlled, phase 3 trial. Lancet. 2023;402:705–19.
6. Drucker DJ. Evolving concepts and translational relevance of enteroendocrine cell biology. J Clin Endocrinol Metab. 2016;101:778–86.
7. Papamargaritis D, le Roux CW. Do gut hormones contribute to weight loss and glycaemic outcomes after bariatric surgery? Nutrients. 2021;13(3):762.
8. Baggio LL, Drucker DJ. Glucagon-like peptide-1 receptor co-agonists for treating metabolic disease. Mol Metab. 2021;46:101090.
9. Christensen MB, Gasbjerg LS, Heimbürger SM, Stensen S, Vilsbøll T, Knop FK. GIP's involvement in the pathophysiology of type 2 diabetes. Peptides. 2020;125:170178.
10. Zhang Q, Delessa CT, Augustin R, Bakhti M, Colldén G, Drucker DJ, et al. The glucose-dependent insulinotropic polypeptide (GIP) regulates body weight and food intake via CNS-GIPR signaling. Cell Metab. 2021;33:833–844.e5.
11. Knop FK, Urva S, Rettinganti M, Benson C, Roell W, Mather KJ, et al. 56-OR: A long-acting glucose dependent insulinotropic polypeptide receptor agonist shows weight loss without nausea or vomiting. Abstract from the 83rd American Diabetes Association meeting. Diabetes. 2023;72. https://doi.org/10.2337/db23-56-OR.
12. Gault VA, Kerr BD, Harriott P, Flatt PR. Administration of an acylated GLP-1 and GIP preparation provides added beneficial glucose-lowering and insulinotropic actions over single incretins in mice with type 2 diabetes and obesity. Clin Sci. 2011;121:107–17.
13. Nørregaard PK, Deryabina MA, Tofteng Shelton P, Fog JU, Daugaard JR, Eriksson PO, et al. A novel GIP analogue, ZP4165, enhances glucagon-like peptide-1-induced body weight loss and improves glycaemic control in rodents. Diabetes Obes Metab. 2018;20:60–8.
14. Finan B, Ma T, Ottaway N, Müller TD, Habegger KM, Heppner KM, et al. Unimolecular dual incretins maximize metabolic benefits in rodents, monkeys, and humans. Sci Transl Med. 2013;5:209ra151.
15. Bergmann NC, Gasbjerg LS, Heimbürger SM, Krogh LSL, Dela F, Hartmann B, et al. No acute effects of exogenous glucose-dependent insulinotropic polypeptide on energy intake, appetite, or energy expenditure when added to treatment with a long-acting glucagon-like peptide 1 receptor agonist in men with type 2 diabetes. Diabetes Care. 2020;43:588–96.
16. Bergmann NC, Lund A, Gasbjerg LS, Meessen ECE, Andersen MM, Bergmann S, et al. Effects of combined GIP and GLP-1 infusion on energy intake, appetite and energy expenditure in overweight/obese individuals: a randomised, crossover study. Diabetologia. 2019;62:665–75.
17. Jastreboff AM, Aronne LJ, Ahmad NN, Wharton S, Connery L, Alves B, et al. Tirzepatide once weekly for the treatment of obesity. N Engl J Med. 2022;387:205–16.
18. Garvey WT, Frias JP, Jastreboff AM, le Roux CW, Sattar N, Aizenberg D, et al. Tirzepatide once weekly for the treatment of obesity in people with type 2 diabetes (SURMOUNT-2): a double-blind, randomised, multicentre, placebo-controlled, phase 3 trial. Lancet. 2023;402:613–26.

19. Boylan MO, Glazebrook PA, Tatalovic M, Wolfe MM. Gastric inhibitory polypeptide immunoneutralization attenuates development of obesity in mice. Am J Physiol Endocrinol Metab. 2015;309:E1008–18.
20. Fulurija A, Lutz TA, Sladko K, Osto M, Wielinga PY, Bachmann MF, et al. Vaccination against GIP for the treatment of obesity. PLoS One. 2008;3:e3163.
21. Killion EA, Lu SC, Fort M, Yamada Y, Véniant MM, Lloyd DJ. Glucose-dependent insulinotropic polypeptide receptor therapies for the treatment of obesity, do agonists = antagonists? Endocr Rev. 2020;41:bnz002.
22. Lu SC, Chen M, Atangan L, Killion EA, Komorowski R, Cheng Y, et al. GIPR antagonist antibodies conjugated to GLP-1 peptide are bispecific molecules that decrease weight in obese mice and monkeys. Cell Rep Med. 2021;2:100263.
23. Strande JL, Kurra V, Jeswani R, Oberoi R, Sharpsten L, Neutel J, et al. A Phase 1, Randomized, double-blind, placebo-controlled single and multipleascending dose study of AMG 133 in subjects with obesity. Metabolism. 2023;142:155433.
24. Le Roux C, Steen O, Lucas KJ, Startseva E, Unseld A, Hennige AM. 51-OR: A Phase 2, Randomized, Double-blind, Placebo-controlled, Dose-finding Study of BI 456906 in people with overweight/obesity. Abstract from the 83rd American Diabetes Association meeting 2023. Diabetes. 2023;72. https://doi.org/10.2337/db23-51-OR.
25. Ji L, Jiang H, Cheng Z, Qiu W, Liao L, Zhang Y, et al. A phase 2 randomised controlled trial of mazdutide in Chinese overweight adults or adults with obesity. Nature. Communications. 2023;14:1–10.
26. Klein S, Nestor JJ, Harris MS, Suyundikov A, Casper R, Steele SM, et al. 334-OR: Pemvidutide (ALT-801), a Balanced (1:1) GLP-1/Glucagon dual receptor agonist, induces rapid and marked weight loss without the need for dose titration in people with overweight/obesity. Abstracts from the 2022 American Diabetes Association Meeting. Diabetes. 2022;71 https://doi.org/10.2337/db22-334-OR.
27. Alba M, Yee J, Frustaci ME, Samtani MN, Fleck P. Efficacy and safety of glucagon-like peptide-1/glucagon receptor co-agonist JNJ-64565111 in individuals with obesity without type 2 diabetes mellitus: a randomized dose-ranging study. Clin Obes. 2021;11:e12432.
28. Di Prospero NA, Yee J, Frustaci ME, Samtani MN, Alba M, Fleck P. Efficacy and safety of glucagon-like peptide-1/glucagon receptor co-agonist JNJ-64565111 in individuals with type 2 diabetes mellitus and obesity: a randomized dose-ranging study. Clin Obes. 2021;11:e12433.
29. Coskun T, Urva S, Roell WC, Qu H, Loghin C, Moyers JS, et al. LY3437943, a novel triple glucagon, GIP, and GLP-1 receptor agonist for glycemic control and weight loss: from discovery to clinical proof of concept. Cell Metab. 2022;34:1234–1247.e9.
30. Jastreboff AM, Kaplan LM, Frías JP, Wu Q, Du Y, Gurbuz S, et al. Triple–hormone-receptor agonist retatrutide for obesity — a phase 2 trial. N Engl J Med. 2023;389:514–26.
31. Rosenstock J, Frias J, Jastreboff AM, Du Y, Lou J, Gurbuz S, et al. Retatrutide, a GIP, GLP-1 and glucagon receptor agonist, for people with type 2 diabetes: a randomised, double-blind, placebo and active-controlled, parallel-group, phase 2 trial conducted in the USA. Lancet. 2023;402:529–44.
32. Boccia L, Gamakharia S, Coester B, Whiting L, Lutz TA, Le Foll C. Amylin brain circuitry. Peptides. 2020;132:170366.
33. Dehestani B, Stratford NRS, le Roux CW. Amylin as a future obesity treatment. J Obes Metab Syndr. 2021;30:320–5.
34. Hay DL, Chen S, Lutz TA, Parkes DG, Roth JD. Amylin: pharmacology, physiology, and clinical potential. Pharmacol Rev. 2015;67:564–600.
35. Smith SR, Aronne LJ, Burns CM, Kesty NC, Halseth AE, Weyer C. Sustained weight loss following 12-month pramlintide treatment as an adjunct to lifestyle intervention in obesity. Diabetes Care. 2008;31:1816.
36. Lau DCW, Erichsen L, Francisco AM, Satylganova A, le Roux CW, McGowan B, et al. Once-weekly cagrilintide for weight management in people with overweight and obesity: a mul-

ticentre, randomised, double-blind, placebo-controlled and active-controlled, dose-finding phase 2 trial. Lancet. 2021;398:2160–72.

37. Enebo LB, Berthelsen KK, Kankam M, Lund MT, Rubino DM, Satylganova A, et al. Safety, tolerability, pharmacokinetics, and pharmacodynamics of concomitant administration of multiple doses of cagrilintide with semaglutide 2·4 mg for weight management: a randomised, controlled, phase 1b trial. Lancet. 2021;397:1736–48.
38. Frias JP, Deenadayalan S, Erichsen L, Knop FK, Lingvay I, Macura S, et al. Efficacy and safety of co-administered once-weekly cagrilintide 2·4 mg with once-weekly semaglutide 2·4 mg in type 2 diabetes: a multicentre, randomised, double-blind, active-controlled, phase 2 trial. Lancet. 2023;402:720–30.
39. Neary NM, Small CJ, Druce MR, Park AJ, Ellis SM, Semjonous NM, et al. Peptide YY3-36 and glucagon-like peptide-17-36 inhibit food intake additively. Endocrinology. 2005;146:5120–7.
40. Sloth B, Davidsen L, Holst JJ, Flint A, Astrup A. Effect of subcutaneous injections of PYY1-36 and PYY3-36 on appetite, ad libitum energy intake, and plasma free fatty acid concentration in obese males. Am J Physiol Endocrinol Metab. 2007;293:E604–9.
41. Batterham RL, Cohen MA, Ellis SM, Le Roux CW, Withers DJ, Frost GS, et al. Inhibition of food intake in obese subjects by peptide YY3-36. N Engl J Med. 2003;349:941–8.
42. Gantz I, Erondu N, Mallick M, Musser B, Krishna R, Tanaka WK, et al. Efficacy and safety of intranasal peptide YY3-36 for weight reduction in obese adults. J Clin Endocrinol Metab. 2007;92:1754–7.
43. Tan TMM, Minnion J, Khoo B, Ball LJ, Malviya R, Day E, et al. Safety and efficacy of an extended-release peptide YY analogue for obesity: a randomized, placebo-controlled, phase 1 trial. Diabetes Obes Metab. 2021;23:1471–83.
44. Heymsfield SB, Coleman LA, Miller R, Rooks DS, Laurent D, Petricoul O, et al. Effect of bimagrumab vs. placebo on body fat mass among adults with type 2 diabetes and obesity: a phase 2 randomized clinical trial. JAMA Netw Open. 2021;4:e2033457.
45. Benichou O, Coskun T, Gonciarz MD, Garhyan P, Adams AC, Du Y, et al. Discovery, development, and clinical proof of mechanism of LY3463251, a long-acting GDF15 receptor agonist. Cell Metab. 2023;35:274–286.e10.
46. Papamargaritis D, le Roux CW, Holst JJ, Davies MJ. New therapies for obesity. Cardiovasc Res. 2022;
47. Kang JG, Park CY. Anti-obesity drugs: a review about their effects and safety. Diabetes Metab J. 2012;36:13–25. https://doi.org/10.4093/dmj.2012.36.1.13.
48. Hill JO. Understanding and addressing the epidemic of obesity: an energy balance perspective. Endocr Rev. 2006;27:750–61. https://doi.org/10.1210/er.2006-0032.
49. Cone RD. Studies on the physiological functions of the melanocortin system. Endocr Rev. 2006;27:736–49. https://doi.org/10.1210/er.2006-0034.
50. Cone RD. Anatomy and regulation of the central melanocortin system. Nat Neurosci. 2005;8:571–8.
51. Chen KY, Muniyappa R, Abel BS, Mullins KP, Staker P, Brychta RJ, et al. RM-493, a melanocortin-4 receptor (MC4R) agonist, increases resting energy expenditure in obese individuals. J Clin Endocrinol Metab. 2015;100:1639–45. https://doi.org/10.1210/jc.2014-4024.
52. Release, O. P. I. P. Orexigen (R) Therapeutics phase 2b trial for Empatic(TM) meets primary efficacy endpoint demonstrating significantly greater weight loss versus comparators in obese patients. http://ir.orexigen.com/phoenix.zhtml%3Fc=207034%26p=irol-newsArticle%26ID=1336796%26highlight=. Accessed 13 Sept 2017.
53. Blundell J, et al. Effects of once-weekly semaglutide on appetite, energy intake, control of eating, food preference and body weight in subjects with obesity. Diabetes Obes Metab. 2017;19:1242–51. https://doi.org/10.1111/dom.12932. The aim of this trial was to investigate the mechanism of action of body weight loss with semaglutide, a new drug which has shown significant weight loss potential of almost 16% in clinical trials.

54. Ravussin E, Smith SR, Mitchell JA, et al. Enhanced weight loss with pramlintide/metreleptin: an integrated neurohormonal approach to obesity pharmacotherapy. Obesity. 2009;17(9):1736–43.
55. Kim DD, Krishnarajah J, Lillioja S, de Looze F, Marjason J, Proietto J, et al. Efficacy and safety of beloranib for weight loss in obese adults: a randomized controlled trial. Diabetes Obes Metab. 2015;17:566–72. https://doi.org/10.1111/dom.12457.
56. Hansen HH, Jensen MM, Overgaard A, Weikop P, Mikkelsen JD. Tesofensine induces appetite suppression and weight loss with reversal of low forebrain dopamine levels in the diet-induced obese rat. Pharmacol Biochem Behav. 2013;110:265–71. https://doi.org/10.1016/j.pbb.2013.07.018.
57. Fisher FM, et al. Obesity is a fibroblast growth factor 21 (FGF21)-resistant state. Diabetes. 2010;59:2781–9. https://doi.org/10.2337/db10-0193.
58. Altabas V, Zjacic-Rotkvic V. Anti-ghrelin antibodies in appetite suppression: recent advances in obesity pharmacotherapy. Immunotargets Ther. 2015;4:123–30. https://doi.org/10.2147/ITT.S60398.
59. Colon-Gonzalez F, Kim GW, Lin JE, Valentino MA, Waldman SA. Obesity pharmacotherapy: what is next? Mol Asp Med. 2013;34:71–83. https://doi.org/10.1016/j.mam.2012.10.005.
60. Takagi K, Legrand R, Asakawa A, Amitani H, François M, Tennoune N, et al. Anti-ghrelin immunoglobulins modulate ghrelin stability and its orexigenic effect in obese mice and humans. Nat Commun. 2013;4:2685. https://doi.org/10.1038/ncomms3685.
61. Svoboda M, Tastenoy M, Vertongen P, Robberecht P. Relative quantitative analysis of glucagon receptor mRNA in rat tissues. Mol Cell Endocrinol. 1994;105(2):131–7.
62. Fonseca VA, Alvarado-Ruiz R, Raccah D, et al. Efficacy and safety of the once-daily GLP-1 receptor agonist lixisenatide in monotherapy: a randomized, double-blind, placebo-controlled trial in patients with type 2 diabetes (GetGoal-Mono). Diabetes Care. 2012;35(6):1225–31.
63. Pfeffer MA, Claggett B, Diaz R, et al. Lixisenatide in patients with type 2 diabetes and acute coronary syndrome. N Engl J Med. 2015;373(23):2247–57.
64. Buchwald H, Estok R, Fahrbach K, et al. Weight and type 2 diabetes after bariatric surgery: systematic review and meta-analysis. Am J Med. 2009;122(3):248–56.e5.
65. Chang SH, Stoll CRT, Song J, Varela JE, Eagon CJ, Colditz GA. The effectiveness and risks of bariatric surgery: an updated systematic review and meta-analysis, 2003–2012. JAMA Surg. 2014;149(3):275–87.
66. Müller TD, Finan B, Clemmensen C, DiMarchi RD, Tschöp MH. The new biology and pharmacology of glucagon. Physiol Rev. 2017;97(2):721–66.
67. Day JW, Ottaway N, Patterson JT, et al. A new glucagon and GLP-1 co-agonist eliminates obesity in rodents. Nat Chem Biol. 2009;5(10):749–57.
68. Nahra R, Wang T, Gadde KM, et al. Effects of cotadutide on metabolic and hepatic parameters in adults with overweight or obesity and type 2 diabetes: a 54-week randomized phase 2b study. Diabetes Care. 2021;44(6):1433–42.
69. Ji L, Gao L, Jiang H, et al. Safety and efficacy of a GLP-1 and glucagon receptor dual agonist mazdutide (IBI362) 9 mg and 10 mg in Chinese adults with overweight or obesity: a randomised, placebo-controlled, multiple-ascending-dose phase 1b trial. eClin Med. 2022;54:101691.
70. Mroz PA, Finan B, Gelfanov V, et al. Optimized GIP analogs promote body weight lowering in mice through GIPR agonism not antagonism. Mol Metab. 2019;20:51–62.
71. Liskiewicz A, Khalil A, Liskiewicz D, et al. Glucose-dependent insulinotropic polypeptide regulates body weight and food intake via GABAergic neurons in mice. Nat Metab. 2023;5(12):2075–85.
72. Frias JP, Bastyr EJ, Vignati L, et al. The sustained effects of a dual GIP/GLP-1 receptor agonist, NNC0090-2746, in patients with type 2 diabetes. Cell Metab. 2017;26(2):343–52.e2.
73. Martin-Rodriguez E, Guillen-Grima F, Marti A, Brugos-Larumbe A. Comorbidity associated with obesity in a large population: the APNA study. Obes Res Clin Pract. 2015;9(5):435–47.

74. Sirtori A, Brunani A, Capodaglio P, Berselli ME, Villa V, Ceriani F, et al. Patients with obesity-related comorbidities have higher disability compared with those without obesity-related comorbidities: results from a cross-sectional study. Int J Rehabil Res. 2016;39(1):63–9.
75. Knowler WC, Barrett-Connor E, Fowler SE, Hamman RF, Lachin JM, Walker EA, et al. Reduction in the incidence of type 2 diabetes with lifestyle intervention or metformin. N Engl J Med. 2002;346(6):393–403.
76. Lean ME, Leslie WS, Barnes AC, et al. Primary care-led weight management for remission of type 2 diabetes (DiRECT): an open-label, cluster-randomised trial. Lancet. 2018;391(10120):541–51.
77. Lindstrom J, Louheranta A, Mannelin M, Rastas M, Salminen V, Eriksson J, et al. The Finnish Diabetes Prevention Study (DPS): lifestyle intervention and 3-year results on diet and physical activity. Diabetes Care. 2003;26(12):3230–6.
78. Zaccardi F, Webb DR, Htike ZZ, Youssef D, Khunti K, Davies MJ. Efficacy and safety of sodium-glucose co-transporter-2 inhibitors in type 2 diabetes mellitus: systematic review and network meta-analysis. Diabetes Obes Metab. 2016;18(8):783–94.
79. Monami M, Nardini C, Mannucci E. Efficacy and safety of sodium glucose co-transport-2 inhibitors in type 2 diabetes: a meta-analysis of randomized clinical trials. Diabetes Obes Metab. 2014;16(5):457–66.
80. Merovci A, Solis-Herrera C, Daniele G, Eldor R, Fiorentino TV, Tripathy D, et al. Dapagliflozin improves muscle insulin sensitivity but enhances endogenous glucose production. J Clin Invest. 2014;124(2):509–14.
81. Liu XY, Zhang N, Chen R, Zhao JG, Yu P. Efficacy and safety of sodium-glucose cotransporter 2 inhibitors in type 2 diabetes: a meta-analysis of randomized controlled trials for 1 to 2years. J Diabetes Complicat. 2015;29(8):1295–303.
82. Maruthur NM, Tseng E, Hutfless S, Wilson LM, Suarez-Cuervo C, Berger Z, et al. Diabetes medications as monotherapy or metformin-based combination therapy for type 2 diabetes: a systematic review and meta-analysis. Ann Intern Med. 2016;164(11):740–51.
83. Mearns ES, Sobieraj DM, White CM, Saulsberry WJ, Kohn CG, Doleh Y, et al. Comparative efficacy and safety of antidiabetic drug regimens added to metformin monotherapy in patients with type 2 diabetes: a network meta-analysis. PLoS One. 2015;10(4):e0125879.
84. Cai X, Yang W, Gao X, Chen Y, Zhou L, Zhang S, et al. The association between the dosage of SGLT2 inhibitor and weight reduction in type 2 diabetes patients: a meta-analysis. Obesity. 2018;26(1):70–80.
85. Ferrannini G, Hach T, Crowe S, Sanghvi A, Hall KD, Ferrannini E. Energy balance after sodium-glucose cotransporter 2 inhibition. Diabetes Care. 2015;38(9):1730–5.
86. Leibel RL, Rosenbaum M, Hirsch J. Changes in energy expenditure resulting from altered body weight. N Engl J Med. 1995;332:621–8.
87. Lundkvist P, Pereira MJ, Katsogiannos P, Sjostrom CD, Johnsson E, Eriksson JW. Dapagliflozin once daily plus exenatide once weekly in obese adults without diabetes: sustained reductions in bodyweight, glycaemia, and blood pressure over 1 year. Diabetes Obes Metab. 2017;
88. Lundkvist P, Sjostrom CD, Amini S, Pereira MJ, Johnsson E, Eriksson JW. Dapagliflozin once-daily and exenatide once-weekly dual therapy: a 24-week randomized, placebo-controlled, phase II study examining effects on body weight and prediabetes in obese adults without diabetes. Diabetes Obes Metab. 2017;19(1):49–60.
89. Neal B, Perkovic V, Mahaffey KW, de Zeeuw D, Fulcher G, Erondu N, et al. Canagliflozin and cardiovascular and renal events in type 2 diabetes. N Engl J Med. 2017;377(7):644–57.
90. Zinman B, Wanner C, Lachin JM, Fitchett D, Bluhmki E, Hantel S, et al. Empagliflozin, cardiovascular outcomes, and mortality in type 2 diabetes. N Engl J Med. 2015;373(22):2117–28.
91. Wiviott SD, Raz I, Bonaca MP, Mosenzon O, Kato ET, Cahn A, et al. Dapagliflozin and cardiovascular outcomes in type 2 diabetes. N Engl J Med. 2019;380:347–57.
92. Rajasekeran H, Lytvyn Y, Cherney DZ. Sodium-glucose cotransporter 2 inhibition and cardiovascular risk reduction in patients with type 2 diabetes: the emerging role of natriuresis. Kidney Int. 2016;89(3):524–6.

93. Mudaliar S, Alloju S, Henry RR. Can a shift in fuel energetics explain the beneficial cardiorenal outcomes in the EMPA-REG OUTCOME study? A unifying hypothesis. Diabetic Care. 2016;39(7):1115–22.
94. Zelniker TA, Wiviott SD, Raz I, Im K, Goodrich EL, Bonaca MP, et al. SGLT2 inhibitors for primary and secondary prevention of cardiovascular and renal outcomes in type 2 diabetes: a systematic review and meta-analysis of cardiovascular outcome trials. Lancet. 2019;393(10166):31–9.
95. Busch RS, Kane MP. Combination SGLT2 inhibitor and GLP-1 receptor agonist therapy: a complementary approach to the treatment of type 2 diabetes. Postgrad Med. 2017;129(7):686–97.
96. Oliva RV, Bakris GL. Blood pressure effects of sodium-glucose co-transport 2 (SGLT2) inhibitors. J Am Soc Hypertens. 2014;8(5):330–9.
97. Sjostrom CD, Hashemi M, Sugg J, Ptaszynska A, Johnsson E. Dapagliflozin-induced weight loss affects 24-week glycated haemoglobin and blood pressure levels. Diabetes Obes Metab. 2015;17(8):809–12.
98. Lambers Heerspink HJ, de Zeeuw D, Wie L, Leslie B, List J. Dapagliflozin a glucose-regulating drug with diuretic properties in subjects with type 2 diabetes. Diabetes Obes Metab. 2013;15(9):853–62.
99. Sano M. A new class of drugs for heart failure: sGLT2 inhibitors reduce sympathetic overactivity. J Cardiol. 2018;71(5):471–6.
100. Hall JE, do Carmo JM, da Silva AA, Wang Z, Hall ME. Obesity-induced hypertension: interaction of neurohumoral and renal mechanisms. Circ Res. 2015;116(6):991–1006.
101. Seidu S, Kunutsor SK, Cos X, Gillani S, Khunti K, For et al. SGLT2 inhibitors and renal outcomes in type 2 diabetes with or without renal impairment: a systematic review and meta-analysis. Prim Care Diabetes 2018;12(3):265–283.
102. Bays HE, Weinstein R, Law G, Canovatchel W. Canagliflozin: effects in overweight and obese subjects without diabetes mellitus. Obesity (Silver Spring). 2014;22(4):1042–9.
103. Henry RR, Thakkar P, Tong C, Polidori D, Alba M. Efficacy and safety of Canagliflozin, a sodium-glucose cotransporter 2 inhibitor, as add-on to insulin in patients with type 1 diabetes. Diabetes Care. 2015;38(12):2258–65.
104. Dandona P, Mathieu C, Phillip M, Hansen L, Griffen SC, Tschope D, et al. Efficacy and safety of dapagliflozin in patients with inadequately controlled type 1 diabetes (DEPICT-1): 24 week results from a multicentre, double-blind, phase 3, randomised controlled trial. Lancet Diabetes Endocrinol. 2017;5(11):864–76.
105. Garg SK, Henry RR, Banks P, Buse JB, Davies MJ, Fulcher GR, et al. Effects of sotagliflozin added to insulin in patients with type 1 diabetes. N Engl J Med. 2017;377(24):2337–48.
106. Vasilakou D, Karagiannis T, Athanasiadou E, Mainou M, Liakos A, Bekiari E, et al. Sodium-glucose cotransporter 2 inhibitors for type 2 diabetes: a systematic review and meta-analysis. Ann Intern Med. 2013;159(4):262–74.
107. Ryan P, Schuemie M, De Falco F, Yuan Z, Stang P et al. Canagliflozin versus other antihyperglycaemic agents on the risk of below-knee amputation for patients with type 2 diabetes: a real world analysis of>700,000 US patients. EASD 54th Annual Meeting 2018; http://abstractsonline.com/pp8/#!/4612/presentation/41802018.
108. Pereira MJ, Lundkvist P, Kamble PG, Lau J, Martins JG, Sjostrom CD, et al. A randomized controlled trial of Dapagliflozin plus once-weekly exenatide versus placebo in individuals with obesity and without diabetes: metabolic effects and markers associated with bodyweight loss. Diabet Ther. 2018;9(4):1511–32.
109. Frias JP, Nauck MA, Van J, Kutner ME, Cui X, Benson C, et al. Efficacy and safety of LY3298176, a novel dual GIP and GLP-1 receptor agonist, in patients with type 2 diabetes: a randomised, placebo-controlled and active comparator-controlled phase 2 trial. Lancet. 2018;
110. Piazza PV, Cota D, Marsicano G. The CB1 receptor as the cornerstone of exostasis. Neuron. 2017;93:1252–74.

111. Quarta C, Mazza R, Obici S, Pasquali R, Pagotto U. Energy balance regulation by endocannabinoids at central and peripheral levels. Trends Mol Med. 2011;17:518–26.
112. Mazier W, Saucisse N, Gatta-Cherifi B, Cota D. The endocannabinoid system: pivotal orchestrator of obesity and metabolic disease. Trends Endocrinol Metab. 2015;26:524–37.
113. Gatta-Cherifi B, Matias I, Vallée M, Tabarin A, Marsicano G, Piazza PV, et al. Simultaneous postprandial deregulation of the orexigenic endocannabinoid anandamide and the anorexigenic peptide YY in obesity. Int J Obes. 2012;36:880–5.
114. Monteleone P, Piscitelli F, Scognamiglio P, Monteleone AM, Canestrelli B, Di Marzo V, et al. Hedonic eating is associated with increased peripheral levels of ghrelin and the endocannabinoid 2-arachidonoyl-glycerol in healthy humans: a pilot study. J Clin Endocrinol Metab. 2012;97:E917–24.
115. Monteleone AM, Di Marzo V, Aveta T, Piscitelli F, Dalle Grave R, Scognamiglio P, et al. Deranged endocannabinoid responses to hedonic eating in underweight and recently weight-restored patients with anorexia nervosa. Am J Clin Nutr. 2015;101:262–9.
116. Fanelli F, Mezzullo M, Belluomo I, Di Lallo VD, Baccini M, Ibarra Gasparini D, et al. Plasma 2-arachidonoylglycerol is a biomarker of age and menopause related insulin resistance and dyslipidemia in lean but not in obese men and women. Mol Metab. 2017;6:406–15.
117. Rinaldi-Carmona M, Barth F, Héaulme M, Shire D, Calandra B, Congy C, et al. SR141716A, a potent and selective antagonist of the brain cannabinoid receptor. FEBS Lett. 1994;350:240–4.
118. Foll BL, Forget B, Aubin H-J, Goldberg SR. Blocking cannabinoid CB1 receptors for the treatment of nicotine dependence: insights from pre-clinical and clinical studies. Addict Biol. 2008;13:239–52.
119. Després J-P, Golay A, Sjöström L, Rimonabant in Obesity-Lipids Study Group. Effects of rimonabant on metabolic risk factors in overweight patients with dyslipidemia. N Engl J Med. 2005;353:2121–34.
120. Després JP, Ross R, Boka G, Alméras N, Lemieux I, ADAGIO-Lipids Investigators. Effect of rimonabant on the high-triglyceride/ low-HDL-cholesterol dyslipidemia, intraabdominal adiposity, and liver fat: the ADAGIO-Lipids trial. Arterioscler Thromb Vasc Biol. 2009;29:416–23.
121. Hollander PA, Amod A, Litwak LE, Chaudhari U, ARPEGGIO Study Group. Effect of rimonabant on glycemic control in insulin-treated type 2 diabetes: the ARPEGGIO trial. Diabetes Care. 2010;33:605–7.
122. Pi-Sunyer FX, Aronne LJ, Heshmati HM, Devin J, Rosenstock J, RIO-North America Study Group. Effect of rimonabant, a cannabinoid-1 receptor blocker, on weight and cardiometabolic risk factors in overweight or obese patients: RIO-North America: a randomized controlled trial. JAMA. 2006;295(7):761–75.
123. Scheen AJ, Finer N, Hollander P, Jensen MD, Van Gaal LF. Efficacy and tolerability of rimonabant in overweight or obese patients with type 2 diabetes: a randomised controlled study. Lancet. 2006;368:1660–72.
124. Christensen R, Kristensen PK, Bartels EM, Bliddal H, Astrup A. Efficacy and safety of the weight-loss drug rimonabant: a meta-analysis of randomised trials. Lancet. 2007;370:1706–13. https://doi.org/10.1016/S0140-6736(07)61721-8.
125. Tam J, Cinar R, Liu J, Godlewski G, Wesley D, Jourdan T, et al. Peripheral cannabinoid-1 receptor inverse agonism reduces obesity by reversing leptin resistance. Cell Metab. 2012;16:167–79.
126. Liu J, Godlewski G, Jourdan T, Liu Z, Cinar R, Xiong K, et al. Cannabinoid-1 receptor antagonism improves glycemic control and increases energy expenditure through sirtuin-1/mechanistic target of RAPAMYCIN complex 2 and 5'adenosine monophosphate-activated protein kinase signaling. Hepatology. 2019;69:1535–48.
127. Cinar R, Godlewski G, Liu J, Tam J, Jourdan T, Mukhopadhyay B, et al. Hepatic cannabinoid-1 receptors mediate diet-induced insulin resistance by increasing de novo synthesis of long-chain ceramides. Hepatology. 2014;59:143–53.

128. Udi S, Hinden L, Ahmad M, Drori A, Iyer MR, Cinar R, et al. Dual inhibition of cannabinoid-1 receptor and iNOS attenuates obesity-induced chronic kidney disease. Br J Pharmacol. 2019; https://doi.org/10.1111/bph.14849.
129. Cinar R, Iyer MR, Liu Z, Cao Z, Jourdan T, Erdelyi K, et al. Hybrid inhibitor of peripheral cannabinoid-1 receptors and inducible nitric oxide synthase mitigates liver fibrosis. JCI Insight. 2016;1:e87336.
130. Matthews JM, McNally JJ, Connolly PJ, Xia M, Zhu B, Black S, et al. Tetrahydroindazole derivatives as potent and peripherally selective cannabinoid-1 (CB1) receptor inverse agonists. Bioorg Med Chem Lett. 2016;26:5346–9.
131. Liu J, Zhou L, Xiong K, Godlewski G, Mukhopadhyay B, Tam J, et al. Hepatic cannabinoid receptor-1 mediates diet-induced insulin resistance via inhibition of insulin signaling and clearance in mice. Gastroenterology. 2012;142:1218–28.e1.
132. Lynn B, Gee A, Zhang L, Pfaus JG. Effects of cannabinoids on female sexual function. Sex Med Rev. 2020;8:18–27.
133. Pacher P, Mukhopadhyay P, Mohanraj R, Godlewski G, Bátkai S, Kunos G. Modulation of the endocannabinoid system in cardiovascular disease. Hypertension. 2008;52:601–7.
134. Christou GA, Katsiki N, Blundell J, Fruhbeck G, Kiortsis DN. Semaglutide as a promising antiobesity drug. Obes Rev. 2019;20:805–15.
135. Müller TD, Clemmensen C, Finan B, DiMarchi RD, Tschöp MH. Anti-obesity therapy: from rainbow pills to polyagonists. Pharmacol Rev. 2018;70:712–46.
136. Quarta C, Clemmensen C, Zhu Z, Yang B, Joseph SS, Lutter D, et al. Molecular integration of incretin and glucocorticoid action reverses immunometabolic dysfunction and obesity. Cell Metab. 2017;26:620–32.e6.
137. Soeliman FA, Azadbakht L. Weight loss maintenance: a review on dietary related strategies. J Res Med Sci. 2014;19:268–75.
138. Huang XF, Yu Y, Beck EJ, South T, Li Y, Batterham MJ, et al. Diet high in oat β-glucan activates the gut-hypothalamic (PYY3-36-NPY) axis and increases satiety in diet-induced obesity in mice. Mol Nutr Food Res. 2011;55:1118–21. https://doi.org/10.1002/mnfr.201100095.
139. Rios-Hoyo A, Gutierrez-Salmean G. New dietary supplements for obesity: what we currently know. Curr Obes Rep. 2016;5:262–70. https://doi.org/10.1007/s13679-016-0214-y.
140. Rahar S, Swami G, Nagpal N, Nagpal MA, Singh GS. Preparation, characterization, and biological properties of beta-glucans. J Adv Pharm Technol Res. 2011;2:94–103. https://doi.org/10.4103/2231-4040.82953.
141. Stohs SJ. Safety, efficacy, and mechanistic studies regarding citrus aurantium (bitter orange) extract and p-synephrine. Phytother Res. 2017;31:1463–74. https://doi.org/10.1002/ptr.5879.
142. Rupasinghe HP, Sekhon-Loodu S, Mantso T, Panayiotidis MI. Phytochemicals in regulating fatty acid beta-oxidation: potential underlying mechanisms and their involvement in obesity and weight loss. Pharmacol Ther. 2016;165:153–63. https://doi.org/10.1016/j.pharmthera.2016.06.005.
143. Stohs SJ, Preuss HG, Shara M. The safety of Citrus aurantium (bitter orange) and its primary protoalkaloid p-synephrine. Phytother Res. 2011;25:1421–8. https://doi.org/10.1002/ptr.3490.
144. Jordan MA. Chapter 4: Interactions of drugs and dietary supplements used for weight loss. In: El-Shemy HA, editor. Drug discovery. Croatia: InTech; 2013. p. 107–55. https://doi.org/10.5772/51145.
145. Harpaz E, Tamir S, Weinstein A, Weinstein Y. The effect of caffeine on energy balance. J Basic Clin Physiol Pharmacol. 2017;28:1–10. https://doi.org/10.1515/jbcpp-2016-0090.
146. Yen M, Ewald MB. Toxicity of weight loss agents. J Med Toxicol. 2012;8:145–52. https://doi.org/10.1007/s13181-012-0213-7.
147. Ngondi JL, Etoundi BC, Nyangono CB, Mbofung CM, Oben JE. IGOB131, a novel seed extract of the West African plant Irvingia gabonensis, significantly reduces body weight and improves metabolic parameters in overweight humans in a randomized double-blind pla-

cebo controlled investigation. Lipids Health Dis. 2009;8:7. https://doi.org/10.1186/1476-511X-8-7.
148. Parikh SJ, Yanovski JA. Calcium intake and adiposity. Am J Clin Nutr. 2003;77:281–7. https://doi.org/10.1093/ajcn/77.2.281.
149. Christensen R, Lorenzen JK, Svith CR, Bartels EM, Melanson EL, Saris WH, et al. Effect of calcium from dairy and dietary supplements on faecal fat excretion: a meta-analysis of randomized controlled trials. Obes Rev. 2009;10:475–86. https://doi.org/10.1111/j.1467-789X.2009.00599.x.
150. Booth AO, Huggins CE, Wattanapenpaiboon N, Nowson CA. Effect of increasing dietary calcium through supplements and dairy food on body weight and body composition: a meta-analysis of randomised controlled trials. Br J Nutr. 2015;114:1013–25. https://doi.org/10.1017/S0007114515001518.
151. Li P, Fan C, Lu Y, Qi K. Effects of calcium supplementation on body weight: a meta-analysis. Am J Clin Nutr. 2016;104:1263–73. https://doi.org/10.3945/ajcn.116.136242.
152. Zheng J, Zheng S, Feng Q, Zhang Q, Xiao X. Dietary capsaicin and its anti-obesity potency: from mechanism to clinical implications. Biosci Rep. 2017:37. https://doi.org/10.1042/BSR20170286.
153. Kang JH, Goto T, Han IS, Kawada T, Kim YM, Yu R. Dietary capsaicin reduces obesity-induced insulin resistance and hepatic steatosis in obese mice fed a high-fat diet. Obesity. 2010;18:780–7. https://doi.org/10.1038/oby.2009.301.
154. Kim J, Park J, Lim K. Nutrition supplements to stimulate lipolysis: a review in relation to endurance exercise capacity. J Nutr Sci Vitaminol. 2016;62:141–61. https://doi.org/10.3177/jnsv.62.141.
155. Pooyandjoo M, Nouhi M, Shab-Bidar S, Djafarian K, Olyaeemanesh A. The effect of (l-) carnitine on weight loss in adults: a systematic review and meta-analysis of randomized controlled trials. Obes Rev. 2016;17:970–6. https://doi.org/10.1111/obr.12436.
156. Hakeshzadeh F, Tabibi H, Ahmadinejad M, Malakoutian T, Hedayati M. Effects of L-carnitine supplement on plasma coagulation and anticoagulation factors in hemodialysis patients. Ren Fail. 2010;32:1109–14. https://doi.org/10.3109/0886022X.2010.510617.
157. Chiu CY, Chan IL, Yang TH, Liu SH, Chiang MT. Supplementation of chitosan alleviates high-fat diet-enhanced lipogenesis in rats via adenosine monophosphate (AMP)-activated protein kinase activation and inhibition of lipogenesis-associated genes. J Agric Food Chem. 2015;63:2979–88. https://doi.org/10.1021/acs.jafc.5b00198.
158. Jull AB, Ni Mhurchu C, Bennett DA, Dunshea-Mooij CA, Rodgers A. Chitosan for overweight or obesity. Cochrane Database Syst Rev. 2008:CD003892. https://doi.org/10.1002/14651858.CD003892.pub3.
159. Pokhis K, Bitterlich N, Cornelli U, Cassano G. Efficacy of polyglucosamine for weight loss-confirmed in a randomized double-blind, placebo-controlled clinical investigation. BMC Obes. 2015;2(25) https://doi.org/10.1186/s40608-015-0053-5.
160. Hua Y, Clark S, Ren J, Sreejayan N. Molecular mechanisms of chromium in alleviating insulin resistance. J Nutr Biochem. 2012;23:313–9. https://doi.org/10.1016/j.jnutbio.2011.11.001.
161. Tian H, Guo X, Wang X, He Z, Sun R, Ge S, et al. Chromium picolinate supplementation for overweight or obese adults. Cochrane Database Syst Rev. 2013:CD010063. https://doi.org/10.1002/14651858.CD010063.pub2.
162. Pittler MH, Stevinson C, Ernst E. Chromium picolinate for reducing body weight: meta-analysis of randomized trials. Int J Obes Relat Metab Disord. 2003;27:522–9. https://doi.org/10.1038/sj.ijo.0802262.
163. Lukaski HC, Siders WA, Penland JG. Chromium picolinate supplementation in women: effects on body weight, composition, and iron status. Nutrition. 2007;23:187–95. https://doi.org/10.1016/j.nut.2006.12.001.
164. Han LK, Morimoto C, Yu RH, Okuda H. Effects of Coleus forskohlii on fat storage in ovariectomized rats. Yakugaku Zasshi. 2005;125:449–53.

165. Godard MP, Johnson BA, Richmond SR. Body composition and hormonal adaptations associated with forskolin consumption in overweight and obese men. Obes Res. 2005;13:1335–43. https://doi.org/10.1038/oby.2005.162.
166. Loftus HL, Astell KJ, Mathai ML, Su XQ. Coleus forskohlii extract supplementation in conjunction with a hypocaloric diet reduces the risk factors of metabolic syndrome in overweight and obese subjects: a randomized controlled trial. Nutrients. 2015;7:9508–22. https://doi.org/10.3390/nu7115483.
167. Virgona N, Taki Y, Yamada S, Umegaki K. Dietary Coleus forskohlii extract generates dose-related hepatotoxicity in mice. J Appl Toxicol. 2013;33:924–32. https://doi.org/10.1002/jat.2770.
168. Lehnen TE, da Silva MR, Camacho A, Marcadenti A, Lehnen AM. A review on effects of conjugated linoleic fatty acid (CLA) upon body composition and energetic metabolism. J Int Soc Sports Nutr. 2015;12:36. https://doi.org/10.1186/s12970-015-0097-4.
169. Plourde M, Jew S, Cunnane SC, Jones PJ. Conjugated linoleic acids: why the discrepancy between animal and human studies? Nutr Rev. 2008;66:415–21. https://doi.org/10.1111/j.1753-4887.2008.00051.x.
170. Onakpoya IJ, Posadzki PP, Watson LK, Davies LA, Ernst E. The efficacy of long-term conjugated linoleic acid (CLA) supplementation on body composition in overweight and obese individuals: a systematic review and meta-analysis of randomized clinical trials. Eur J Nutr. 2012;51:127–34. https://doi.org/10.1007/s00394-011-0253-9.
171. Wan-Loy C, Siew-Moi P. Marine algae as a potential source for anti-obesity agents. Mar Drugs. 2016:14. https://doi.org/10.3390/md14120222.
172. Saito M, Ueno M, Ogino S, Kubo K, Nagata J, Takeuchi M. High dose of Garcinia cambogia is effective in suppressing fat accumulation in developing male Zucker obese rats, but highly toxic to the testis. Food Chem Toxicol. 2005;43:411–9. https://doi.org/10.1016/j.fct.2004.11.008.
173. Wu MT, Chou HN, Huang CJ. Dietary fucoxanthin increases metabolic rate and upregulated mRNA expressions of the PGC-1alpha network, mitochondrial biogenesis and fusion genes in white adipose tissues of mice. Mar Drugs. 2014;12:964–82. https://doi.org/10.3390/md12020964.
174. Onakpoya I, Hung SK, Perry R, Wider B, Ernst E. The use of garcinia extract (hydroxycitric acid) as a weight loss supplement: a systematic review and meta-analysis of randomised clinical trials. J Obes. 2011;2011:509038. https://doi.org/10.1155/2011/509038.
175. Heymsfield SB, Allison DB, Vasselli JR, Pietrobelli A, Greenfield D, Nunez C. Garcinia cambogia (hydroxycitric acid) as a potential antiobesity agent: a randomized controlled trial. JAMA. 1998;280:1596–600.
176. de Lira-García C, Souto-Gallardo M, Bacardí-Gascón M, Jiménez-Cruz A. A systematic review of the effectiveness of alternative weight-loss products' ingredients. Rev Salud Publ. 2008;10:818–30.
177. Mattes RD, Bormann L. Effects of (−)-hydroxycitric acid on appetitive variables. Physiol Behav. 2000;71:87–94.
178. Gallaher CM, Munion J, Hesslink R Jr, Wise J, Gallaher DD. Cholesterol reduction by glucomannan and chitosan is mediated by changes in cholesterol absorption and bile acid and fat excretion in rats. J Nutr. 2000;130:2753–9. https://doi.org/10.1093/jn/130.11.2753.
179. Sood N, Baker WL, Coleman CI. Effect of glucomannan on plasma lipid and glucose concentrations, body weight, and blood pressure: systematic review and meta-analysis. Am J Clin Nutr. 2008;88:1167–75. https://doi.org/10.1093/ajcn/88.4.1167.
180. Onakpoya I, Posadzki P, Ernst E. The efficacy of glucomannan supplementation in overweight and obesity: a systematic review and meta-analysis of randomized clinical trials. J Am Coll Nutr. 2014;33:70–8. https://doi.org/10.1080/07315724.2014.870013.
181. Butt MS, Shahzadi N, Sharif MK, Nasir M. Guar gum: a miracle therapy for hypercholesterolemia, hyperglycemia and obesity. Crit Rev Food Sci Nutr. 2007;47:389–96. https://doi.org/10.1080/10408390600846267.

182. Rao TP. Role of guar fiber in appetite control. Physiol Behav. 2016;164(Pt A):277–83. https://doi.org/10.1016/j.physbeh.2016.06.014.
183. Komarnytsky S, Esposito D, Poulev A, Raskin I. Pregnane glycosides interfere with steroidogenic enzymes to down-regulate corticosteroid production in human adrenocortical H295R cells. J Cell Physiol. 2013;228:1120–6. https://doi.org/10.1002/jcp.24262.
184. Vermaak I, Hamman JH, Viljoen AM. Hoodia gordonii: an up-to-date review of a commercially important anti-obesity plant. Planta Med. 2011;77:1149–60. https://doi.org/10.1055/s-0030-1250643.
185. Blom WA, Abrahamse SL, Bradford R, Duchateau GS, Theis W, Orsi A, et al. Effects of 15-d repeated consumption of Hoodia gordonii purified extract on safety, ad libitum energy intake, and body weight in healthy, overweight women: a randomized controlled trial. Am J Clin Nutr. 2011;94:1171–81. https://doi.org/10.3945/ajcn.111.020321.
186. Onakpoya I, Davies L, Posadzki P, Ernst E. The efficacy of Irvingia gabonensis supplementation in the management of overweight and obesity: a systematic review of randomized controlled trials. J Diet Suppl. 2013;10:29–38. https://doi.org/10.3109/19390211.2012.760508.
187. Ross AC, Manson JE, Abrams SA, Aloia JF, Brannon PM, Clinton SK, et al. The 2011 report on dietary reference intakes for calcium and vitamin D from the Institute of Medicine: what clinicians need to know. J Clin Endocrinol Metab 2011;96:53–58. https://doi.org/10.1210/jc.2010-2704
188. EFSA. Scientific Opinion on the substantiation of a health claim related to a standardised aqueous extract from white kidney bean (Phaseolus vulgaris L.) and reduction of body weight pursuant to Article 13(5) of Regulation (EC) No 1924/20061. EFSA Panel on Dietetic Products, Nutrition and Allergies (NDA). EFSA J. 2014;12:3754. www.efsa.europa.eu/efsajournal.
189. Udani J, Tan O, Molina J. Systematic review and meta-analysis of a proprietary alpha-amylase inhibitor from white bean (Phaseolus vulgaris L.) on weight and fat loss in humans. Food Secur. 2018;7:E63. https://doi.org/10.3390/foods7040063.
190. Koh-Banerjee PK, Ferreira MP, Greenwood M, Bowden RG, Cowan PN, Almada AL, et al. Effects of calcium pyruvate supplementation during training on body composition, exercise capacity, and metabolic responses to exercise. Nutrition. 2005;21:312–9. https://doi.org/10.1016/j.nut.2004.06.026.
191. Leu SY, Chen YC, Tsai YC, Hung YW, Hsu CH, Lee YM, et al. Raspberry ketone reduced lipid accumulation in 3T3-L1 cells and ovariectomy-induced obesity in wistar rats by regulating autophagy mechanisms. J Agric Food Chem. 2017;65:10907–14. https://doi.org/10.1021/acs.jafc.7b03831.
192. Lopez HL, Ziegenfuss TN, Hofheins JE, Habowski SM, Arent SM, Weir JP, et al. Eight weeks of supplementation with a multi-ingredient weight loss product enhances body composition, reduces hip and waist girth, and increases energy levels in overweight men and women. J Int Soc Sports Nutr. 2013;10:22–35. https://doi.org/10.1186/1550-2783-10-22.
193. Pal S, Ellis V. The chronic effects of whey proteins on blood pressure, vascular function, and inflammatory markers in overweight individuals. Obesity. 2010;18:1354–9.
194. Fekete AA, Giromini C, Chatzidiakou Y, Givens DI, Lovegrove JA. Whey protein lowers blood pressure and improves endothelial function and lipid biomarkers in adults with prehypertension and mild hypertension: results from the chronic Whey2Go randomized controlled trial. Am J Clin Nutr. 2016;104:1534–44.
195. Pal S, Ellis V, Dhaliwal S. Effects of whey protein isolate on body composition, lipids, insulin and glucose in overweight and obese individuals. Br J Nutr. 2010;104:716–23.
196. Baer DJ, Stote KS, Paul DR, Harris GK, Rumpler WV, Clevidence BA. Whey protein but not soy protein supplementation alters body weight and composition in free-living overweight and obese adults. J Nutr. 2011;141:1489–94.
197. McGregor RA, Poppitt SD. Milk protein for improved metabolic health: a review of the evidence. Nutr Metab. 2013;10:46.

198. Lattimer JM, Haub MD. Effects of dietary fiber and its components on metabolic health. Nutrients. 2010;2:1266–89.
199. Freeland KR, Wilson C, Wolever TMS. Adaptation of colonic fermentation and glucagon-like peptide-1 secretion with increased wheat fibre intake for 1 year in hyperinsulinaemic human subjects. Br J Nutr. 2009;103:82–90.
200. Lu ZX, Walker KZ, Muir JG, O'Dea K. Arabinoxylan fibre improves metabolic control in people with type II diabetes. Eur J Clin Nutr. 2004;58:621–8.
201. Rakvaag E, Fuglsang-Nielsen R, Bach Knudsen KE, Landberg R, Johannesson Hjelholt A, Søndergaard E, et al. Whey protein combined with low dietary fiber improves lipid profile in subjects with abdominal obesity: a randomized, controlled trial. Nutrients. 2019;11:2091.
202. Weickert MO, Roden M, Isken F, Hoffmann D, Nowotny P, Osterhoff M, et al. Effects of supplemented isoenergetic diets differing in cereal fiber and protein content on insulin sensitivity in overweight humans. Am J Clin Nutr. 2011;94:459–71.
203. Kim KS, Jang MJ, Fang S, et al. Anti-obesity effect of taurine through inhibition of adipogenesis in white fat tissue but not in brown fat tissue in a high-fat diet-induced obese mouse model. Amino Acids. 2019;51(2):245–54. https://doi.org/10.1007/s00726-018-2659-7.
204. Guo YY, Li BY, Peng WQ, et al. Taurine-mediated browning of white adipose tissue is involved in its anti-obesity effect in mice. J Biol Chem. 2019;294(41):15014–24. https://doi.org/10.1074/jbc.RA119.009936.
205. Goodpaster BH, Sparks LM. Metabolic flexibility in health and disease. Cell Metab. 2017;25(5):1027–36. https://doi.org/10.1016/j.cmet.2017.04.015.
206. Leal LG, Lopes MA, Batista ML. Physical exercise-induced myokines and muscle-adipose tissue crosstalk: a review of current knowledge and the implications for health and metabolic diseases. Front Physiol. 2018;9:1307. https://doi.org/10.3389/fphys.2018.01307.
207. Batitucci G, Brandao CFC, De Carvalho FG, et al. Taurine supplementation increases irisin levels after high intensity physical training in obese women. Cytokine. 2019;123:154741. https://doi.org/10.1016/j.cyto.2019.154741.
208. De Carvalho FG, Brandao CFC, Batitucci G, et al. Taurine supplementation associated with exercise increases mitochondrial activity and fatty acid oxidation gene expression in the subcutaneous white adipose tissue of obese women. Clin Nutr. 2021;40:2180–7. https://doi.org/10.1016/j.clnu.2020.09.044.
209. Rosa FT, Freitas EC, Deminice R, et al. Oxidative stress and inflammation in obesity after taurine supplementation: a double-blind, placebo-controlled study. Eur J Nutr. 2014;53(3):823–30. https://doi.org/10.1007/s00394-013-0586-7.
210. Flegal KM, Wei R, Ogden C. Weight-for-stature compared with body mass index–for-age growth charts for the United States from the Centers for Disease Control and Prevention. Am J Clin Nutr. 2002;75(4):761–6.
211. Boyer BP, Nelson JA, Holub SC. Childhood body mass index trajectories predicting cardiovascular risk in adolescence. J Adolesc Health. 2015;56(6):599–605.
212. Baker JL, Olsen LW, Sørensen TI. Childhood body-mass index and the risk of coronary heart disease in adulthood. N Engl J Med. 2007;357(23):2329–37.
213. Baños RM, Cebolla A, Botella C, García-Palacios A, Oliver E, Zaragoza I, et al. Improving childhood obesity treatment using new technologies: the ETIOBE system. Clin Pract Epidemiol Mental Health. 2011;7:62.
214. Santos HO, Lavie CJ. Weight loss and its influence on high-density lipoprotein cholesterol (HDL-C) concentrations: a noble clinical hesitation. Clin Nutr ESPEN. 2021;42:90–2.
215. Santos HO, Macedo RC. Impact of intermittent fasting on the lipid profile: assessment associated with diet and weight loss. Clin Nutr ESPEN. 2018;24:14–21.
216. Field AE, Austin S, Taylor C, Malspeis S, Rosner B, Rockett HR, et al. Relation between dieting and weight change among preadolescents and adolescents. Pediatrics. 2003;112(4):900–6.
217. Fisher JO, Birch LL. Restricting access to foods and children's eating. Appetite. 1999;32(3):405–19.

218. Fisher JO, Birch LL. Restricting access to palatable foods affects children's behavioral response, food selection, and intake. Am J Clin Nutr. 1999;69(6):1264–72.
219. Kirby M, Danner E. Nutritional deficiencies in children on restricted diets. Pediatr Clin. 2009;56(5):1085–103.
220. García OP, Long KZ, Rosado JL. Impact of micronutrient deficiencies on obesity. Nutr Rev. 2009;67(10):559–72.
221. Papathanasopoulos A, Camilleri M. Dietary fiber supplements: effects in obesity and metabolic syndrome and relationship to gastrointestinal functions. Gastroenterology. 2010;138(1):65–72 e2.
222. Kimm SY. The role of dietary fiber in the development and treatment of childhood obesity. Pediatrics. 1995;96(5):1010–4.
223. Saltzman E, Moriguti JC, Das SK, Corrales A, Fuss P, Greenberg AS, Roberts SB. Effects of a cereal rich in soluble fiber on body composition and dietary compliance during consumption of a hypocaloric diet. J Am Coll Nutr. 2001;20(1):50–7.
224. Jovanovski EMN, Komishon A, Khayyat R, Li D, Blanco Mejia S, Khan T, Jenkins AL, Smircic-Duvnjak L, Sievenpiper JL, Vuksan V. Can dietary viscous fiber affect body weight independently of an energy-restrictive diet? A systematic review and meta-analysis of randomized controlled trials. Am J Clin Nutr. 2019;111:471–85.
225. Kim SJ, de Souza RJ, Choo VL, Ha V, Cozma AI, Chiavaroli L, Mirrahimi A, Blanco Mejia S, Di Buono M, Bernstein AM, Leiter LA, Kris-Etherton PM, Vuksan V, Beyene J, Kendall CW, Jenkins DJ, Sievenpiper JL. Effects of dietary pulse consumption on body weight: a systematic review and meta-analysis of randomized controlled trials. Am J Clin Nutr. 2016;103(5):1213–23. https://doi.org/10.3945/ajcn.115.124677.
226. Australian Bureau of Statistics. Australian health survey: consumption of food groups from the Australian dietary guidelines. Canberra: ABS; 2016.
227. Pal S, Khossousi A, Binns C, Dhaliwal S, Ellis V. The effect of a fibre supplement compared to a healthy diet on body composition, lipids, glucose, insulin and other metabolic syndrome risk factors in overweight and obese individuals. Br J Nutr. 2011;105(1):90–100.
228. Anderson JW, Baird P, Davis RH Jr, Ferreri S, Knudtson M, Koraym A, et al. Health benefits of dietary fiber. Nutr Rev. 2009;67(4):188–205.
229. Solah VA, Kerr DA, Hunt WJ, Johnson SK, Boushey CJ, Delp EJ, et al. Effect of fibre supplementation on body weight and composition, frequency of eating and dietary choice in overweight individuals. Nutrients. 2017;9(2):149.
230. Pal S, Ho S, Gahler RJ, Wood S. Effect on body weight and composition in overweight/obese Australian adults over 12 months consumption of two different types of fibre supplementation in a randomized trial. Nutr Metab. 2016;13(1):82.
231. Pal S, Radavelli-Bagatini S. Effects of psyllium on metabolic syndrome risk factors. Obes Rev. 2012;13(11):1034–47.
232. Delzenne NM, Cani PD, Everard A, Neyrinck AM, Bindels LB. Gut microorganisms as promising targets for the management of type 2 diabetes. Diabetologia. 2015;58(10):2206–17.
233. Delzenne NM, Olivares M, Neyrinck AM, Beaumont M, Kjolbaek L, Larsen TM, et al. Nutritional interest of dietary fiber and prebiotics in obesity: lessons from the MyNewGut consortium. Clin Nutr. 2020;39(2):414–24.
234. Rodriguez J, Hiel S, Neyrinck AM, Le Roy T, Potgens SA, Leyrolle Q, et al. Discovery of the gut microbial signature driving the efficacy of prebiotic intervention in obese patients. Gut. 2020;69(11):1975–87.
235. Hiel S, Gianfrancesco MA, Rodriguez J, Portheault D, Leyrolle Q, Bindels LB, et al. Link between gut microbiota and health outcomes in inulin -treated obese patients: lessons from the Food4Gut multicenter randomized placebo-controlled trial. Clin Nutr. 2020;39(12):3618–28.
236. Allen JM, Mailing LJ, Niemiro GM, Moore R, Cook MD, White BA, et al. Exercise alters gut microbiota composition and function in lean and obese humans. Med Sci Sports Exerc. 2018;50(4):747–57.

237. Lambert JE, Myslicki JP, Bomhof MR, Belke DD, Shearer J, Reimer RA. Exercise training modifies gut microbiota in normal and diabetic mice. Appl Physiol Nutr Metab. 2015;40(7):749–52.
238. Evans CC, LePard KJ, Kwak JW, Stancukas MC, Laskowski S, Dougherty J, et al. Exercise prevents weight gain and alters the gut microbiota in a mouse model of high fat diet-induced obesity. PLoS One. 2014;9(3):e92193.
239. Campbell SC, Wisniewski PJ, Noji M, McGuinness LR, Haggblom MM, Lightfoot SA, et al. The effect of diet and exercise on intestinal integrity and microbial diversity in mice. PLoS One. 2016;11(3):e0150502.
240. Rios JL, Hart DA, Reimer RA, Herzog W. Prebiotic and exercise do not alter knee osteoarthritis in a rat model of established obesity. Cartilage. 2020; https://doi.org/10.1177/1947603520959399.
241. Melson E, Ashraf U, Papamargaritis D, Davies MJ. What is the pipeline for future medications for obesity? Int J Obes. 2024; https://doi.org/10.1038/s41366-024-01473-y.
242. Srivastava G, Apovian C. Future pharmacotherapy for obesity: new anti-obesity drugs on the horizon. Curr Obes Rep. 2018; https://doi.org/10.1007/s13679-018-0300-4.
243. Gutgesell RM, Nogueiras R, Tschöp MH, Müller TD. Dual and triple incretin-based co-agonists: novel therapeutics for obesity and diabetes. Diabetes Ther. 2024; https://doi.org/10.1007/s13300-024-01566-x.
244. Pereira MJ, Eriksson JW. Emerging role of SGLT-2 inhibitors for the treatment of obesity. Drugs. 2019; https://doi.org/10.1007/s40265-019-1057-0.
245. Quarta C, Cota D. Anti-obesity therapy with peripheral CB1 blockers: from promise to safe(?) practice. Int J Obes. 2020; https://doi.org/10.1038/s41366-020-0577-8.
246. Barrea L, Altieri B, Polese B, De Conno B, Muscogiuri G, Colao A, Savastano S. Nutritionist and obesity: brief overview on efficacy, safety, and drug interactions of the main weight-loss dietary supplements. Int J Obes Suppl. 2019; https://doi.org/10.1038/s41367-019-0007-3.
247. Fuglsang-Nielsen R, Rakvaag E, Langdahl B, Knudsen KE, Hartmann B, Holst JJ, Hermansen K, Gregersen S. Effects of whey protein and dietary fiber intake on insulin sensitivity, body composition, energy expenditure, blood pressure, and appetite in subjects with abdominal obesity. Eur J Clin Nutr. 2020; https://doi.org/10.1038/s41430-020-00759-4.
248. De Carvalho FG, Brandao CF, Muñoz VR, Batitucci G, Tavares ME, Teixeira GR, Pauli JR, De Moura LP, Ropelle ER, Cintra DE, da Silva AS. Taurine supplementation in conjunction with exercise modulated cytokines and improved subcutaneous white adipose tissue plasticity in obese women. Amino Acids. 2021; https://doi.org/10.1007/s00726-021-03041-4.
249. Fatahi S, Sayyari AA, Salehi M, Safa M, Sohouli M, Shidfar F, Santos HO. The effects of chitosan supplementation on anthropometric indicators of obesity, lipid and glycemic profiles, and appetite-regulated hormones in adolescents with overweight or obesity: a randomized, double-blind clinical trial. BMC Pediatr. 2022; https://doi.org/10.1186/s12887-022-03590-x.
250. Jovanovski E, Mazhar N, Komishon A, Khayyat R, Li D, Blanco Mejia S, Khan T, Jenkins AL, Smircic-Duvnjak L, Sievenpiper JL, Vuksan V. Effect of viscous fiber supplementation on obesity indicators in individuals consuming calorie-restricted diets: a systematic review and meta-analysis of randomized controlled trials. Eur J Nutr. 2020; https://doi.org/10.1007/s00394-020-02224-1.
251. Pal S, McKay J, Ho S, Jane M, Gahler RJ, Wood S. Micronutrient status of individuals with overweight and obesity following 3 months' supplementation with PolyGlycopleX (PGX®) or psyllium: a randomized controlled trial. BMC Nutr. 2022; https://doi.org/10.1186/s40795-022-00534-7.
252. Rodriguez J, Neyrinck AM, Van Kerckhoven M, Gianfrancesco MA, Renguet E, Bertrand L, Cani PD, Lanthier N, Cnop M, Paquot N, Thissen J-P, Bindels LB, Delzenne NM. Physical activity enhances the improvement of body mass index and metabolism by inulin: a multicenter randomized placebo-controlled trial performed in obese individuals. BMC Med. 2022; https://doi.org/10.1186/s12916-022-02299-z.

Chapter 7
Person Centered Approach and Challenges in the Management of Obesity

Shilpa Chugh Garcha and Sanjay Kalra

Obesity is a chronic health condition and the management approach generally involves changes in lifestyle and use of pharmacotherapy over long periods. Lifestyle modifications including diet changes and physical activity are the cornerstone of management of obesity. Pharmacological management of obesity is recommended in individuals with a body mass index (BMI) of $\geq$30 kg/m^2 (obese) or a BMI of $\geq$27 kg/m^2 (overweight) with at least one bodyweight-related comorbidity [1].

Conventionally, BMI is used to diagnose and classify obesity and further guide management, however, many approaches have been discussed over time for patient-centric diagnosis of obesity which takes into consideration other factors as well. Some of these are the '4 M approach' by Canadian Obesity Association, the Edmonton Obesity Staging System, Barophynotypic characterization, the SECURED model, and BaroSixer model to set targets in management of obesity [2].

The selection of an anti-obesity medication for an individual depends on various factors. The presence of co-morbidities such as diabetes mellitus, underlying liver disease and others play a crucial role in decision-making along with other factors including adverse effects associated with medications, route of administration, and their economic implications.

One of the studies included explores the use of anti-obesity medications (AOMs) based on their added benefits when used for weight management. The study explores the role of various AOMs in the management of obesity with associated comorbidities such as type 2 diabetes, cardiovascular disease, obstructive sleep apnea, non-alcoholic fatty liver disease, osteoarthritis, and others and how this approach can

S. C. Garcha (✉)
Sonepat, Haryana, India

S. Kalra
Department of Endocrinology, Bharti Hospital, Karnal, Haryana, India

S. C. Garcha, S. Kalra (eds.), *Drugs for Medical Management of Obesity*,
https://doi.org/10.1007/978-981-96-1651-0_7

help in better individualization of the treatment and a step towards precision medicine in obesity.

One specific study explores the impact of different obesity management strategies or various anti-obesity medications on cardiovascular risk factors and outcomes. It provides a comprehensive review of the available data which can guide clinical decision-making.

Specific eating behaviors are an important underlying cause of obesity and one of the studies included explores the role of various AOMs that affect the food intake, satiety, and reward behavior through their central action. The study included medications such as liraglutide, bupropion/naltrexone, phentermine/topiramate, and lorcaserin (discontinued now).

Another important topic is antipsychotic-induced obesity as the use of some antipsychotics especially second-generation antipsychotics has been associated with weight gain and other metabolic events. One of the studies mentioned here explores the effects of topiramate and metformin on obesity in patients with schizophrenia or affective disorder and who are stable on second-generation antipsychotics. Another study, a double-blind randomized controlled pilot trial studied the impact of liraglutide in overweight or obese individuals with schizophrenia, schizoaffective disorder, or first-episode psychosis.

Introduction of newer molecules for the management of obesity has helped in improving the management of obesity, however, at the same time this has raised concerns regarding the associated adverse events as there has been some drug withdrawals due to associated serious adverse events. Many molecules have recently been approved and it would be important to look for their efficacy and safety in the real world. Clinical decision-making would also depend on their adverse event profile. One of the studies included is a retrospective analysis carried out to identify and characterize adverse events associated with AOMs over long periods.

Childhood obesity is on the rise and it may be due to various underlying factors including genetic and environmental and is associated with an increased risk of comorbidities. The management of obesity needs to be individualized as per the specific needs of the children and adolescents as compared to the adults. Some of the approved AOMs are also approved for use in pediatric age group. One of the studies included delves into the area of biological predisposition towards specific body-weight set point and role of biological and developmental factors along with an obesogenic environment. The study explores the role of comprehensive treatment including lifestyle changes, AOMs and/or metabolic surgery and the efficacy, safety, and tolerability of AOMs in pediatric age group.

Literature also suggests the off-label use of some medications in the management of obesity. Medications approved for use in conditions other than obesity, when used for weight loss, then their use is considered as off-label. One of the studies mention the off-label options including metformin, zonisamide and canagliflozin and the importance of evidence-based use of off-label drugs.

Two studies mentioned in this chapter explore the off-label use of metformin which is one of the first-line drugs used in the management of type 2 diabetes mellitus. One of the studies reviewed the literature to understand the multiple pathways through which metformin acts and how these contribute to its anorexigenic action. Another study is a meta-analysis of randomized controlled trials that compared the various dosages of metformin in overweight adults without diabetes and underscored the importance of dose optimization of metformin for weight loss in different age groups and how its efficacy may be different in adolescents and adults. This study suggests that metformin can lower body mass index at optimal doses and lifestyle modifications along with play an important role in this health condition.

Topiramate is another medication that is being used as an off-label agent. As per one of the studies included, the combination of phentermine/topiramate which is approved by the USFDA was aimed to reduce the prenatal exposure to topiramate, however, an increase in topiramate use was seen after the approval of this combination which may undermine the risk-mitigation efforts and it is important to further explore the risk of accidental prenatal exposures with topiramate when used for this unapproved indication.

Pramlintide, a synthetic amylin analogue is a subcutaneous injectable medication approved for use in the management of type 1 and type 2 diabetes. One of the studies included explores the effect of pramlintide on weight loss and revealed that it increased satiety and decreased total energy intake suggesting it to be an effective treatment for the management of obesity.

Many new molecules have been approved by the regulatory bodies in the last few years making a long list of drugs available now for the management of obesity. This large armamentarium of approved and off-label medications presents many options for managing obesity but also makes it challenging for the physician to select the most appropriate medications as per the individual needs and associated health conditions.

References for Introduction

1. Apovian CM, Aronne LJ, Bessesen DH, McDonnell ME, Murad MH, Pagotto U, Ryan DH, Still CD. Pharmacological management of obesity: an endocrine society clinical practice guideline. J Clin Endocrinol Metab 2015;100(2):342–362. https://doi.org/10.1210/jc.2014-3415
2. Kalra S, Kapoor N, Kota S, Das S. Person-centred obesity care—techniques, thresholds, tools and targets. Eur Endocrinol 2020;16(1):11–3. https://doi.org/10.17925/EE.2020.16.1.11

7.1 Machine Generated Summaries

Disclaimer: The summaries in this chapter were generated from Springer Nature publications using abstractive AI auto-summarization: An abstraction-based summarizer creates new text based on deep learning. New phrases are created to summarize the content. As the constituted sentences are machine selected, they may not fully reflect the body of the work, so we strongly advise that the original content is read and cited. The auto-generated summaries were curated by the editor to meet Springer Nature publication standards.

Machine generated keywords: metformin, antiobesity medication, topiramate, weight gain, liraglutide, antiobesity, management obesity

Effectiveness of Anti-obesity Medications Approved for Long-Term Use in a Multidisciplinary Weight Management Program: A Multi-center Clinical Experience [139]

This is a machine-generated summary of:

Caldefron, Gerardo; Gonzalez-Izundegui, Daniel; Shan, Kuangda L.; Garcia-Valencia, Oscar A.; Cifuentes, Lizeth; Campos, Alejandro; Collazo-Clavell, Maria L.; Shah, Meera; Hurley, Daniel L.; Abu Lebdeh, Haitham S.; Sharma, Mayank; Schmitz, Kristine; Clark, Matthew M.; Grothe, Karen; Mundi, Manpreet S.; Camilleri, Michael; Abu Dayyeh, Barham K.; Hurtado Andrade, Maria D.; Mokadem, Mohamad A.; Acosta, Andres: Effectiveness of anti-obesity medications approved for long-term use in a multidisciplinary weight management program: a multi-center clinical experience [139]

Published in: International Journal of Obesity (2021)

Link to original: https://doi.org/10.1038/s41366-021-01019-6

If you want to cite the papers, please refer to the original.

For technical reasons we could not place the page where the original quote is coming from.

Research highlights

Introduction:

Obesity has emerged as a significant health crisis, with over one-third of US adults classified as obese, leading to increased risks for various diseases and substantial economic costs. Despite lifestyle modifications being the primary intervention for weight management, their effectiveness is often limited. Now a new study by Gerardo Calderon et al. addresses the efficacy of anti-obesity medications (AOMs) in real-world clinical settings, providing insights into their long-term use and associated outcomes.

Main Body:

Calderon's team conducted a retrospective multi-site study across three multidisciplinary weight management clinics, examining patient records from January 2016 to January 2020. The study included patients with a BMI $\geq$30 kg/m^2 or $\geq$ 27 kg/m^2 with comorbidities who were prescribed FDA-approved AOMs for long-term use. Exclusion criteria, omitted those with prior weight loss surgery or endoscopic interventions or inability to afford medications. The researchers utilized a comprehensive review of electronic medical records to gather data on weight loss outcomes and side effects.

The primary endpoint was the percentage of total body weight loss (%TBWL) over 2 years. Secondary endpoints included proportion of patients with body weight reduction from baseline of $\geq$5%, $\geq$10%, $\geq$15%, and $\geq$20%, changes in health status including lipids, glycemic indices, and blood pressure from baseline, and weight regain after medication discontinuation. Statistical analyses incorporated multiple regression and logistic regression to identify factors influencing %TBWL.

Conclusion:

The study revealed significant weight loss at various intervals up to 24 months, with maximum %TBWL observed at 24 months. Discontinuation of AOMs led to weight regain up to 95–96%, highlighting the need for sustained treatment. Phentermine/topiramate-ER emerged as the most effective medication for weight loss at 12 months but also had a higher incidence of adverse events. The research underscores the potential of AOMs in clinical practice, aligning with results from randomized clinical trials (RCTs). However, Calderon et al. emphasize the necessity for careful monitoring due to the high frequency of side effects and call for future research to optimize AOM efficacy and tolerance.

Beyond Weight Loss: Added Benefits Could Guide the Choice of Anti-obesity Medications [140]

This is a machine-generated summary of:

Guglielmi, Valeria; Bettini, Silvia; Sbraccia, Paolo; Busetto, Luca; Pellegrini, Massimo; Yumuk, Volkan; Colao, Anna Maria; El Ghoch, Marwan; Muscogiuri, Giovanna: Beyond Weight Loss: Added Benefits Could Guide the Choice of Anti-Obesity Medications [140]

Published in: Current Obesity Reports (2023)

Link to original: https://doi.org/10.1007/s13679-023-00502-7

If you want to cite the papers, please refer to the original.

For technical reasons we could not place the page where the original quote is coming from.

Research highlights

Introduction:

Obesity is a multifaceted health issue that not only shortens life expectancy but also contributes to a range of comorbidities, including type 2 diabetes and various psychological, neurological, pulmonary, and musculoskeletal diseases. This places a significant financial strain on healthcare systems. Despite advancements in obesity treatment options, the prevalence of obesity continues to rise, indicating a gap in our understanding of effective management strategies. Current medications in Europe for obesity management include orlistat, liraglutide, and the combination of naltrexone hydrochloride/bupropion HCl. Now a new study by Valeria Guglielmi et al. addresses the need for tailored obesity treatments by reviewing evidence on centrally-acting anti-obesity drugs and considering conventional comorbidities to provide more precise patient-tailored treatment options.

Main Body:

Guglielmi et al.'s research delves into the efficacy and safety of existing drugs like naltrexone/bupropion and liraglutide, as well as upcoming medications such as semaglutide, cagrilintide, and tirzepatide. The study meticulously examines the mechanisms by which these drugs suppress appetite and promote weight loss. For instance, naltrexone/bupropion's synergistic effect on the hypothalamus reduces appetite and increases self-control over eating impulses. The authors also explore how liraglutide's GLP-1 receptor agonism leads to insulin secretion and satiety without significant hypoglycemia risk.

The paper further investigates the impact of these drugs on various obesity-related conditions including type 2 diabetes, cardiovascular disease, non-alcoholic fatty liver disease, obstructive sleep apnea, neurodegenerative diseases, depression, and osteoarthritis. Semaglutide's role in reducing food intake with minimal effects on energy expenditure is highlighted alongside its ability to access brain regions involved in food intake regulation. The study also considers the potential additive effects of combining semaglutide with cagrilintide for improved weight control.

Conclusion:

The main advances presented by Guglielmi et al. include a comprehensive analysis of how centrally-acting anti-obesity drugs can be used to optimize treatment based on individual patient comorbidities, moving towards a precision medicine approach in obesity management. The authors suggest that future research should continue to explore the heterogeneity among patients with obesity to achieve better weight loss responses through phenotype-guided interventions. As quoted by Guglielmi, "The evolving scenario of the availability of anti-obesity drugs and the increasing knowledge of their added effects on obesity complications will allow clinicians to move into a new era of precision medicine." This research highlights not only the metabolic and cardiovascular benefits but also less explored clinical advantages and potential drawbacks of these medications, paving the way for more personalized and effective obesity treatments.

Obesity Management in Cardiometabolic Disease: State of the Art [141]

This is a machine-generated summary of:

Iwamoto, Sean J.; Abushamat, Layla A.; Zaman, Adnin; Millard, Anthony J.; Cornier, Marc-Andre: Obesity Management in Cardiometabolic Disease: State of the Art [141]

Published in: Current Atherosclerosis Reports (2021)
Link to original: https://doi.org/10.1007/s11883-021-00953-0

If you want to cite the papers, please refer to the original.

For technical reasons we could not place the page where the original quote is coming from.

Research highlights

Introduction:

The escalating prevalence of obesity worldwide poses a critical challenge to public health, with the condition being intricately linked to numerous comorbidities that compromise nearly every organ system. Particularly concerning is the impact of obesity on cardiovascular disease (CVD), where it stands as an independent risk factor for adverse cardiovascular events. Despite various interventions such as lifestyle modification, pharmacotherapy, and bariatric surgery showing promise in mitigating these risks through weight loss, the extent of weight reduction remains a pivotal determinant in improving CVD outcomes and mortality. Now a new study by Sean J. Iwamoto and colleagues delves into the nuanced effects of different obesity management strategies on cardiovascular risk factors and outcomes, providing a comprehensive review of contemporary data to guide clinical decision-making.

Main Body:

Iwamoto et al.'s narrative review meticulously synthesizes evidence from an array of clinical trials and observational studies to unravel the complex relationship between obesity treatments and cardiometabolic health. The authors underscore the foundational role of lifestyle modifications, including diet, exercise, and behavioral changes, in achieving weight loss and enhancing cardiovascular fitness. They highlight findings from landmark trials such as Look AHEAD and PREDIMED, which demonstrate the differential impacts of intensive lifestyle interventions and dietary patterns on weight loss and CVD risk factors. The study also scrutinizes the efficacy of various FDA-approved anti-obesity medications, revealing their potential in achieving clinically meaningful weight reduction while also drawing attention to their cardiovascular safety profiles. Iwamoto et al.'s analysis extends to endoscopic bariatric therapies and bariatric surgery, with the latter shown to offer substantial long-term benefits for weight loss maintenance and CVD risk reduction.

Conclusion:

The research conducted by Iwamoto et al. represents a significant advance in our understanding of how different obesity management approaches can influence cardiometabolic outcomes. The study reaffirms that while all interventions can improve CVD risk factors to some degree, bariatric surgery stands out for its profound impact on sustained weight loss and improvement in CVD events. The study highlights the importance of individualized treatment strategies for obesity and underscores the need for ongoing research to optimize care for patients with obesity-related cardiometabolic disorders. As we look towards future directions, this comprehensive review sets the stage for more personalized approaches to managing obesity's cardiovascular implications.

Tailoring Pharmacotherapy to Specific Eating Behaviours in Obesity: Can Recommendations for Personalised Therapy Be Made From the Current Data? [142]

This is a machine-generated summary of:

Roberts, Carl A.; Christiansen, Paul; Halford, Jason C. G.: Tailoring pharmacotherapy to specific eating behaviours in obesity: Can recommendations for personalised therapy be made from the current data? [142]

Published in: Acta Diabetologica (2017)

Link to original: https://doi.org/10.1007/s00592-017-0994-x

If you want to cite the papers, please refer to the original.

For technical reasons we could not place the page where the original quote is coming from.

Research highlights

Introduction:

The global obesity pandemic continues to escalate, with the World Health Organization reporting millions of obese individuals within a broader demographic of over a billion overweight adults. This epidemic not only undermines physical and psychological well-being but also imposes substantial economic burdens, as evidenced by the annual costs to the UK's National Health Service and wider economy, amounting to billions of pounds. Now a new study by Carl A. Roberts and colleagues delves into the intricacies of appetite regulation and its implications for personalized pharmacotherapy in obesity management, offering insights into how drug therapy can potentially modify eating behavior and facilitate weight loss.

Main Body:

Roberts et al. provides a comprehensive review of the latest mono and combination pharmacotherapies for obesity, excluding orlistat due to its peripheral action. The study meticulously examines the mechanisms through which these drugs influence satiety, inhibitory control (IC), and reward processes—key factors in appetite regulation that are often compromised in obese individuals. For instance, liraglutide, a glucagon-like peptide-1 receptor agonist, has been shown to reduce food intake and enhance satiety through its action on central pathways. Similarly, the combination therapy of bupropion/naltrexone targets POMC neurons to strengthen satiation signals. The authors also explore lorcaserin's selective serotonin receptor activation to reduce food intake and phentermine/topiramate's synergistic effects on weight loss.

By integrating data from clinical trials with neurophysiological evidence, Roberts et al. shed light on how these drugs may alter eating patterns and pave the way for more targeted obesity treatments.

Conclusion:

The key advances highlighted by Roberts et al.'s study underscore the potential of pharmacotherapy to address behavioral issues associated with obesity by modulating appetite control mechanisms. While promising, the research also points towards the need for more detailed investigations into how these drugs affect specific eating behaviors and their interplay with genetic factors. As per the authors, understanding individual differences in response to pharmacotherapy is crucial for developing personalized treatments. Future research directions include large-scale genetic studies to identify predictors of drug response and tailored interventions based on behavioral risk profiles. This personalized approach could revolutionize obesity treatment by aligning pharmacological strategies with patients' unique physiological and psychological characteristics.

Outcomes and Safety of Concomitant Topiramate or Metformin for Antipsychotics-induced Obesity: A Randomized-Controlled Trial [143]

This is a machine-generated summary of:

Wang, Congjie; Shi, Wenjie; Xu, Jianyang; Huang, Chengbing; Zhu, Jiannan: Outcomes and safety of concomitant topiramate or metformin for antipsychotics-induced obesity: a randomized-controlled trial [143]

Published in: Annals of General Psychiatry (2020)

Link to original: https://doi.org/10.1186/s12991-020-00319-x

If you want to cite the papers, please refer to the original.

For technical reasons we could not place the page where the original quote is coming from.

Research highlights

Introduction:

The use of second-generation antipsychotics (SGAs) has been associated with weight gain and metabolic disturbances, posing significant health risks for patients with psychiatric disorders. Despite various interventions, including pharmacological approaches like orlistat, bupropion, liraglutide, metformin and topiramate, the management of SGA-induced obesity remains a clinical challenge due to inconsistent results and a lack of direct comparative studies. Now a new study by Congjie Wang and colleagues addresses this gap by directly comparing the effects of topiramate and metformin on obesity in patients with schizophrenia or affective disorder, who are stable on SGAs.

Main Body:

Wang's team conducted an open-label randomized clinical trial at Huai'an No. 3 People's Hospital, involving Chinese Han population with patients diagnosed with schizophrenia or affective disorders. The study spanned from September 2012 to December 2016, with participants continuing their original antipsychotic regimen while being randomly assigned to receive either topiramate or metformin. Measurements of weight, height, BMI, waist-hip ratio, and other health indicators were taken every 4 weeks for atleast 16 weeks over the course of the trial. "The aim of this study was to explore the effects of concomitant topiramate or metformin on obesity caused by some SGAs while keeping the patient's illness stable," explains Wang. The researchers ensured rigorous follow-up and data collection protocols to maintain the integrity of their findings.

Conclusion:

The study revealed that topiramate was at least as effective as metformin in managing SGA-induced obesity, demonstrating significant reductions in weight, BMI, and waist-hip ratio over the follow-up period. The study also noted that topiramate showed a faster and more pronounced therapeutic effect on obesity caused by SGAs. While both drugs were well-tolerated with similar safety profiles, topiramate's robust effect suggests it may be a preferable option for weight management in this patient population. Looking forward, Wang emphasizes the need for individualized treatment plans that consider both medication and behavioral interventions for optimal outcomes in managing antipsychotic-induced weight gain.

Liraglutide and the Management of Overweight and Obesity in People with Severe Mental Illness: Qualitative Sub-study [144]

This is a machine-generated summary of:

Barnard-Kelly, Katharine; Whicher, Clare A.; Price, Hermione C.; Phiri, Peter; Rathod, Shanaya; Asher, Carolyn; Peveler, Robert C.; Holt, Richard I. G.: Liraglutide and the management of overweight and obesity in people with severe mental illness: qualitative sub-study [144]

Published in: BMC Psychiatry (2022)

For technical reasons we could not place the page where the original quote is coming from.

Research highlights

Background:

The escalating rates of obesity have become a significant public health concern, with individuals suffering from severe mental illnesses such as schizophrenia or bipolar disorder being particularly vulnerable. These populations experience obesity rates several times higher than the general populace, exacerbating their already heightened risk of morbidity and mortality. While short-term lifestyle interventions have shown some efficacy in weight reduction, their impact remains modest, with a recent meta-analysis by Speyer et al. indicating minimal BMI reduction. Now a new study by Katharine Barnard-Kelly and colleagues addresses this critical issue by exploring the effectiveness of glucagon-like peptide-1 (GLP-1) receptor agonists, specifically liraglutide, in managing obesity among people with severe mental illness.

Main Body:

Barnard-Kelly's team conducted a qualitative sub-study within a double-blind randomized controlled pilot trial to assess the feasibility and impact of daily liraglutide injections on overweight or obese individuals with schizophrenia, schizoaffective disorder, or first episode psychosis. The study spanned from July 2018 to May 2020 at various health centers within the Southern Health NHS Foundation Trust in the UK. Participants were randomized to receive either liraglutide or a placebo and were supported through self-injection training and text reminders. Participants reported clinically relevant weight loss and improved quality of life. The researchers meticulously documented participant experiences and healthcare professional insights through semi-structured interviews, ensuring robust thematic analysis.

Advances and Future Directions:

The study's findings underscore the potential of GLP-1 receptor agonists as a viable treatment for obesity in patients with severe mental illness, offering not just weight loss but also enhanced quality of life. "The intervention could be transformative," suggests Barnard-Kelly, reflecting on participants who described significant improvements in physical mobility and mental well-being. Looking ahead, the research team advocates for further exploration into long-term outcomes and integration into routine care practices. The positive reception from both patients and healthcare providers paves the way for broader application and underscores the need for innovative approaches to tackle obesity within this vulnerable population.

Descriptive Analysis of Reported Adverse Events Associated with Anti-obesity Medications Using FDA Adverse Event Reporting System (FAERS) Databases 2013–2020 [145]

This is a machine-generated summary of:

Alsuhibani, Abdulrahman; Alrasheed, Marwan; Gari, Musaab; Hincapie, Ana L.; Guo, Jeff Jianfei: Descriptive analysis of reported adverse events associated with anti-obesity medications using FDA Adverse Event Reporting System (FAERS) databases 2013–2020 [145]

Published in: International Journal of Clinical Pharmacy (2021)

Link to original: https://doi.org/10.1007/s11096-021-01330-2

If you want to cite the papers, please refer to the original.

For technical reasons we could not place the page where the original quote is coming from.

Research highlights

Background and Key Findings:

Obesity, a condition characterized by excessive body fat accumulation, presents a growing global health crisis, affecting millions and leading to numerous health complications. Despite the long-term strategies of education and environmental and lifestyle modifications to combat obesity, many individuals require pharmacological interventions to achieve significant weight loss. Anti-obesity medications (AOMs), while beneficial in reducing weight, have raised concerns due to serious adverse events (AEs) leading to drug withdrawals from the market. Now a new study by Abdulrahman Alsuhibani and colleagues delves into the characterization of AEs associated with AOMs, utilizing data from the FDA Adverse Event Reporting System (FAERS) to provide a comprehensive analysis of these risks.

Study Narrative:

Alsuhibani's team conducted a retrospective descriptive analysis covering reports from the first quarter of 2013 to the second quarter of 2020. The FAERS database served as a pivotal resource for this study, offering insights into post-marketing safety surveillance. By analyzing all major AE reports linked to six major FDA-approved AOMs (orlistat, lorcaserin, liraglutide, phentermine, phentermine/topiramate, and naltrexone/bupropion) the researchers could categorize AEs by clinical similarity such as cardiovascular, kidney injury, cancers and others and assess outcomes such as life-threatening, hospitalization, requiring intervention, disability and death. The study's methodology was robust, employing SAS Version 9.4 and Microsoft Excel for data analysis. Most reported adverse events were nausea and vomiting followed by dizziness and headache. Notably, cardiovascular and kidney injuries were among the most reported AEs for certain medications like phentermine, phentermine/topiramate and liraglutide. The researchers' approach underscores the importance of pharmacovigilance in understanding the real-world implications of AOM use.

Advances and Future Directions:

The study represents a significant advance in identifying and characterizing AEs associated with AOMs over an extensive period. It highlights that serious cardiovascular and kidney adverse events are not uncommon, emphasizing the need for healthcare providers to monitor AOM utilization closely. Looking forward, this research paves the way for future studies that could compare reported AEs with those listed on official product labels, enhancing our understanding of AOM safety. As Alsuhibani suggests, "The proper use of medication through following the pharmacist's or the physician's instructions can significantly reduce undesirable effects," pointing towards an ongoing need for education around AOM administration to minimize risks effectively.

(Note: This highlight is based on provided text excerpts and may not reflect all aspects of Abdulrahman Alsuhibani's original research paper.)

Current and Future Pharmacotherapies for Obesity in Children and Adolescents [146]

This is a machine-generated summary of:

Kelly, Aaron S.: Current and future pharmacotherapies for obesity in children and adolescents [146]

Published in: Nature Reviews Endocrinology (2023)

Link to original: https://doi.org/10.1038/s41574-023-00858-9

If you want to cite the papers, please refer to the original.

For technical reasons we could not place the page where the original quote is coming from.

Research highlights

Introduction:

Childhood obesity has become a global epidemic, with rates soaring in the wake of the COVID-19 pandemic. This condition, affecting millions, is not merely a transient phase but often persists into adulthood, with over 80% of affected youths retaining their excess weight as they grow older. Obesity in children is linked to a heightened risk of mortality from cardiovascular diseases and type 2 diabetes mellitus. While clinical definitions vary, obesity is typically classified using BMI metrics adjusted for age and sex. Now a new study by Aaron S. Kelly addresses the pressing need for effective interventions by examining the safety, efficacy, and tolerability of novel anti-obesity medications (AOMs) in young populations.

Main Body:

Kelly's study delves into the complex interplay between genetics, environment, and physiology that underpins obesity. The study scrutinizes the 'set point' theory, which suggests that our bodies defend a certain level of adiposity much like a thermostat maintains room temperature. This dynamic makes weight loss particularly challenging for adolescents whose biological and developmental factors further complicate matters. The study evaluated several AOMs, including glucagon-like peptide receptor agonists (liraglutide and semaglutide) and phentermine–topiramate combinations. These medications act on various pathways to reduce appetite, enhance satiety, and diminish food cravings—ultimately aiming to reset the body's defended level of adiposity.

Conclusion:

The study by Kelly marks significant progress in understanding and treating adolescent obesity—a chronic condition demanding sustained intervention. The introduction of AOMs offers a promising avenue for altering physiological processes that have long thwarted weight management efforts. Looking ahead, the research underscores the necessity for ongoing treatment that adapts over time to counteract the body's tenacious defense of its weight set point.

As we anticipate future directions, Kelly emphasizes that the use of AOMs should not be viewed as 'the easy way out' but rather as an essential component in a comprehensive treatment strategy along with lifestyle and behavioral modifications. With several new medications on the horizon, there is hope for more effective management of pediatric obesity that could challenge even the surgical outcomes.

Metformin: Mechanisms in Human Obesity and Weight Loss [147]

This is a machine-generated summary of:

Yerevanian, Armen; Soukas, Alexander A.: Metformin: Mechanisms in Human Obesity and Weight Loss [147]

Published in: Current Obesity Reports (2019)

Link to original: https://doi.org/10.1007/s13679-019-00335-3

If you want to cite the papers, please refer to the original.

For technical reasons we could not place the page where the original quote is coming from.

Research highlights

Introduction:

Since medieval times, extracts from *Galega officinalis*, commonly known as French lilac, have been used for their medicinal properties, including the treatment of diabetes. In the twentieth century, substances related to active ingredients in french lilac, synthetic biguanides such as phenformin, buphormin, and metformin were developed and recognized for their antidiabetic effects. Metformin, in particular, has become a cornerstone in the management of type 2 diabetes due to its safety and efficacy. Now a new study by Armen Yerevanian and Alexander A. Soukas delves into metformin's role beyond glycemic control, exploring its potential in obesity management.

Main Body:

Yerevanian and Soukas comprehensive review examines the multifaceted effects of metformin on weight loss and prevention. Initial studies highlighted modest and variable weight reduction with metformin use. The Diabetes Prevention Study (DPP) substantiated the weight loss findings associated with metformin use by demonstrating sustained weight loss in high-risk individuals adherent to metformin over several years. The authors meticulously dissected various studies to understand how metformin influences weight. They found that while smaller studies yielded inconsistent results on weight loss, larger trials like the DPP showed a clear benefit.

The authors explored various studies to understand metformin's mechanisms of action. They explored its impact on hepatic glucose production, appetite regulation through central nervous system pathways, by influencing gut-brain axis, and gastrointestinal effects that may contribute to its anorexigenic properties. Yerevanian and Soukas also considered the drug's role in altering gut microbiome. This study also explored its potential role in preventing weight gain associated with antipsychotic medications.

Conclusion:

The review by Yerevanian and Soukas marks significant advances in our understanding of metformin's role in obesity management. While not approved as a standalone weight loss medication by the FDA, metformin is increasingly recognized for its benefits in metabolic complications associated with obesity. The authors underscore the importance of continuous research that should continue to unravel the complex interactions between metformin, appetite regulation, central hypothalamic signal, gut microbiota, and incretin secretion. The review suggests that metformin's influence on multiple pathways related to obesity presents new avenues for therapeutic interventions and its impact on aging.

Role of Metformin in Overweight and Obese People Without Diabetes: A Systematic Review and Network Meta-analysis [148]

This is a machine-generated summary of:

Hui, Fuhai; Zhang, Yingshi; Ren, Tianshu; Li, Xiang; Zhao, Mingyi; Zhao, Qingchun: Role of metformin in overweight and obese people without diabetes: a systematic review and network meta-analysis [148]

Published in: European Journal of Clinical Pharmacology (2018)

Link to original: https://doi.org/10.1007/s00228-018-2593-3

Copyright of the summarized publication:

If you want to cite the papers, please refer to the original.

For technical reasons we could not place the page where the original quote is coming from.

Research highlights

Background and Key Findings:

The global obesity crisis poses significant health risks, including heightened cardiovascular and cancer risks. While weight loss can mitigate these dangers, sustaining it remains a challenge. Now a new study by Fuhai Hui et al. addresses this issue through a network meta-analysis, evaluating the efficacy of metformin—a drug primarily used for type 2 diabetes—in aiding weight loss for overweight individuals without diabetes.

Study Narrative:

Fuhai Hui's team conducted a comprehensive review, adhering to rigorous protocols and standards such as PROSPERO, PRISMA, and Cochrane Collaboration guidelines. They included randomized controlled trials (RCTs) that compared various doses and durations of metformin interventions in non-diabetic overweight individuals. The analysis incorporated both direct comparisons between interventions and indirect evidence across studies to estimate the most effective metformin dosage and treatment period. The researchers meticulously assessed the risk of bias using the Physiotherapy Evidence Database scale and evaluated metabolic outcomes alongside weight loss efficacy.

Advances and Future Directions:

The study's findings suggest that metformin can significantly reduce body mass index (BMI) and weight, and dose of 1000 mg/day for adolescents for 3 months and 3000 mg/day and 1000 mg/day for adults may be suitable options along with lifestyle modifications. Notably, metformin was most effective in adolescents compared to adults, where lifestyle changes showed greater efficacy. The research also indicates that metformin does not have a specific effect on lipid and liver metabolism or inflammatory and cardiovascular risk markers. Fuhai Hui's work underscores the need to optimize metformin dosing strategies for weight loss in different age groups while ensuring safety over extended use periods.

Topiramate Utilization after Phentermine/Topiramate Approval for Obesity Management: Risk Minimization in the Era of Drug Repurposing [149]

This is a machine-generated summary of:

Sarayani, Amir; Hampp, Christian; Brown, Joshua D.; Donahoo, William Troy; Winterstein, Almut G.: Topiramate Utilization After Phentermine/Topiramate Approval for Obesity Management: Risk Minimization in the Era of Drug Repurposing [149]

Published in: Drug Safety (2022)
Link to original: https://doi.org/10.1007/s40264-022-01244-6

If you want to cite the papers, please refer to the original.

For technical reasons we could not place the page where the original quote is coming from.

Research highlights

Obesity is a global health concern with limited pharmacological interventions that are both safe and effective. Many drugs like bupropion, topiramate, and liraglutide initially approved for other indications are now repositioned for obesity management. While using the drugs such as topiramte, the challenge remains in balancing efficacy with safety, particularly in vulnerable populations such as women of childbearing potential. Now a new study by Amir Sarayani and colleagues investigates the impact of phentermine/topiramate extended-release approval on the off-label use of topiramate alone for obesity management, considering the risk-benefit profile and regulatory requirements such as Risk Evaluation and Mitigation Strategy (REMS).

The researchers utilized the MarketScan® Commercial Claims Research Databases to conduct an interrupted time-series analysis from January 2009 to December 2015. They focused on new topiramate initiations among individuals with obesity but without other conditions commonly treated with topiramate. The study design accounted for potential confounders like comorbidities and demographic shifts. Sarayani et al. employed segmented regression models to assess changes in prescribing trends before and after the approval of phentermine/topiramate, using metformin and atorvastatin as comparators.

The study revealed a significant increase in topiramate initiation following the approval of phentermine/topiramate, particularly among women without other common indications for topiramate use. This suggests that despite REMS for the combination product aimed at minimizing prenatal exposure to topiramate, there was a notable shift towards using single-ingredient topiramate off-label for obesity management. The authors highlight that this shift could undermine risk mitigation efforts due to less stringent regulatory measures for single-ingredient topiramate compared to the combination product. Future directions include further research into accidental prenatal exposures and indication-specific risk mitigation strategies to optimize patient outcomes while considering the complexities of drug repurposing across different patient populations.

Effect of Pramlintide on Satiety and Food Intake in Obese Subjects and Subjects with Type 2 Diabetes [150]

This is a machine-generated summary of:

Chapman, I.; Parker, B.; Doran, S.; Feinle-Bisset, C.; Wishart, J.; Strobel, S.; Wang, Y.; Burns, C.; Lush, C.; Weyer, C.; Horowitz, M.: Effect of pramlintide on satiety and food intake in obese subjects and subjects with type 2 diabetes [150]

Published in: Diabetologia (2005)
Link to original: https://doi.org/10.1007/s00125-005-1732-4

If you want to cite the papers, please refer to the original.

For technical reasons we could not place the page where the original quote is coming from.

Research highlights

Introduction:

The regulation of food intake and body weight is a complex process involving various peptide hormones that signal satiety and fullness to the central nervous system. While hormones like ghrelin, cholecystokinin, pancreatic polypeptide, and many other hormones have been studied for their roles in this regulatory network, the physiological role of amylin, a peptide hormone co-secreted with insulin, has garnered interest due to its anorexigenic and glucoregulatory effects in animal models. Now a new study by I. Chapman and colleagues addresses the knowledge gap regarding amylin's role in human satiety by examining the effects of pramlintide, a synthetic analogue of amylin, on food intake in humans.

Main Body:

Chapman's team conducted a randomized, double-blind, placebo-controlled crossover study with two distinct groups: subjects with insulin-treated type 2 diabetes and obese subjects without diabetes. The researchers meticulously designed the study to minimize confounding factors, such as excluding females due to menstrual cycle effects on hunger. The primary aim was to test whether pramlintide enhances satiety and reduces ad libitum food intake compared to placebo. Subjects received subcutaneous injections of pramlintide or placebo followed by a standardized preload meal and later an ad libitum buffet meal. The team measured total energy and macronutrient intake using the DIET/4 program and recorded subjective ratings of hunger, fullness, and nausea using visual analogue scales (VAS). Additionally, blood samples were collected to assess postprandial hormonal and metabolic responses.

Conclusion:

The study revealed that pramlintide significantly reduced total energy intake at the buffet meal in both diabetic and obese non-diabetic subjects without affecting macronutrient preference or meal duration. VAS ratings indicated that pramlintide enhanced the satiating effect of meals during both prandial and postprandial periods without increasing nausea. These findings suggest that pramlintide could be an effective treatment for obesity by reducing food intake through enhanced satiety rather than gastrointestinal discomfort (feeling of nausea). Chapman et al.'s research provides valuable insights into amylin's role in human appetite regulation and its therapeutic potential for weight management.

Obesity Pharmacotherapy: A Review of Current Practices and Future Directions [151]

This is a machine-generated summary of:

Schmitz, Sarah; Tchang, Beverly G.; Shukla, Alpana P.: Obesity Pharmacotherapy: a Review of Current Practices and Future Directions [151]

Published in: Current Treatment Options in Gastroenterology (2023)

Link to original: https://doi.org/10.1007/s11938-023-00409-1

If you want to cite the papers, please refer to the original.

For technical reasons we could not place the page where the original quote is coming from.

Research highlights

Introduction:

Obesity, a chronic disease linked to numerous health complications, remains a significant public health challenge worldwide. Despite the known benefits of weight reduction, maintaining long-term weight loss is difficult due to physiological adaptations that increase hunger and lower metabolic rate. Now a new study by Sarah Schmitz and colleagues addresses this challenge by exploring the efficacy of various anti-obesity medications (AOMs) and their potential for long-term obesity management.

Main Body:

Schmitz et al. conducted a comprehensive review of current and emerging AOMs, assessing their mechanisms of action, effectiveness, and safety profiles. The authors highlight that while lifestyle modifications are the cornerstone of obesity treatment, pharmacotherapy can significantly enhance weight loss outcomes. They emphasize the importance of individualizing treatment plans to balance benefits against potential risks. For instance, if a patient does not achieve at least 4–5% weight loss after 12–16 weeks on an AOM, discontinuation is recommended.

The study delves into the specifics of FDA-approved medications like orlistat, phentermine/topiramate, bupropion/naltrexone, liraglutide, gelesis 100, and semaglutide as well as off-label options such as canagliflozin, an SGLT 2 inhibitor, metformin, and zonisamide. Combination therapies are also discussed as a strategy to counteract biological mechanisms that lead to weight regain. Schmitz and her team underscore the need for off-label prescribing to be evidence-informed, especially given the cost barriers associated with many AOMs.

Conclusion:

The key advance from Schmitz et al.'s research is the detailed analysis of both established and novel pharmacotherapies for obesity, offering insights into their relative effectiveness and safety. The study points towards a future where multi-target agents could revolutionize obesity management. As Schmitz notes, "While older AOMs can produce 5–10% weight loss, newer agents can produce 10–15% weight loss." The research suggests that personalized medicine, considering individual patient factors and leveraging combination therapies, will be central to effective long-term obesity management. With several promising medications in development, there is hope for treatments with efficacy nearing that of surgical interventions.

Bibliography

1. Gadde KM, Allison DB, Ryan DH, Peterson CA, Troupin B, Schwiers ML, et al. Effects of low-dose, controlled-release, phentermine plus topiramate combination on weight and associated comorbidities in overweight and obese adults (CONQUER): a randomised, placebo-controlled, phase 3 trial. Lancet. 2011;377:1341–52.
2. Smith SR, Weissman NJ, Anderson CM, Sanchez M, Chuang E, Stubbe S, et al. Multicenter, placebo-controlled trial of lorcaserin for weight management. N Engl J Med. 2010;363(3):245–56.
3. Greenway FL, Fujioka K, Plodkowski RA, Mudaliar S, Guttadauria M, Erickson J, et al. Effect of naltrexone plus bupropion on weight loss in overweight and obese adults (COR-I): a multicentre, randomised, double-blind, placebo-controlled, phase 3 trial. Lancet. 2010;376:595–605.
4. Pi-Sunyer X, Astrup A, Fujioka K, Greenway F, Halpern A, Krempf M, et al. A randomized, controlled trial of 3.0 mg of liraglutide in weight management. N Engl J Med. 2015;373:11–22.
5. Wadden TA, Hollander P, Klein S, Niswender K, Woo V, Hale PM, et al. Weight maintenance and additional weight loss with liraglutide after low-calorie-diet-induced weight loss: the SCALE Maintenance randomized study. Int J Obes. 2013;37(11):1443–51.
6. Astrup A, et al. Safety, tolerability and sustained weight loss over 2 years with the once-daily human GLP-1 analog, liraglutide. Int J Obes. 2012;36:843–54.
7. Garvey WT, Ryan DH, Look M, Gadde KM, Allison DB, Peterson CA, Schwiers M, Day WW, Bowden CH. Two-year sustained weight loss and metabolic benefits with controlled-release phentermine/topiramate in obese and overweight adults (SEQUEL): a randomized, placebo-con-trolled, phase 3 extension study. Am J Clin Nutr. 2012;95:297–308. https://doi.org/10.3945/ajcn.111.024927.
8. Allison DB, Gadde KM, Garvey WT, Peterson CA, Schwiers ML, Najarian T, et al. Controlled-release phentermine/topiramate in severely obese adults: a randomized controlled trial (EQUIP). Obesity. 2012;20:330–42.
9. Gorgojo-Martínez JJ, Basagoiti-Carreño B, Sanz-Velasco A, Serrano-Moreno C, Almodóvar-Ruiz F. Effectiveness and tolerability of orlistat and liraglutide in patients with obesity in a real-world setting: the XENSOR Study. Int J Clin Pract. 2019;73:e13399.
10. Park JH, Kim JY, Choi JH, Park HS, Shin H-Y, Lee JM, et al. Effectiveness of liraglutide 3 mg for the treatment of obesity in a real-world setting without intensive lifestyle intervention. Int J Obes. 2021;45:776–86.
11. Piantanida E, Gallo D, Tanda ML. Liraglutide is an effective drug for the treatment of obesity also in real life. J Endocrinol Investig. 2020;43:1827–8.

12. Wharton S, Liu A, Pakseresht A, Nørtoft E, Haase CL, Mancini J, et al. Real-world clinical effectiveness of liraglutide 3.0 mg for weight management in Canada. Obesity. 2019;27:917–24.
13. Ferrari F, Fierabracci P, Salvetti G, Jaccheri R, Vitti J, Scartabelli G, et al. Weight loss effect of liraglutide in real-life: the experience of a single Italian obesity center. J Endocrinol Investig. 2020;43:1779–85.
14. Fakhreddine AY, Bagsic S, Fujioka K, Frenette CT. Safety and efficacy of pharmacologic weight loss in patients with cirrhosis. Obes Sci Pract. 2021;7:159–67.
15. Ganguly R, Tian Y, Kong SX, Hersloev M, Hobbs T, Smolarz BG, et al. Persistence of newer anti-obesity medications in a real-world setting. Diabetes Res Clin Pract. 2018;143:348–56.
16. Shibuya K, Ali KF, Ji X, Milinoivh A, Bauman J, Kattan MW, et al. The benefit of short-term weight loss with anti-obesity medications in real-world clinical practice. Endocr Pract. 2019;25:1022–8.
17. Elangovan A, Shah R, Smith ZL. Pharmacotherapy for obesity—trends using a population level national database. Obes Surg. 2021;31:1105–12.
18. Apovian CM, Aronne LJ, Bessesen DH, McDonnell ME, Murad MH, Pagotto U, et al. Pharmacological management of obesity: an endocrine society clinical practice guideline. J Clin Endocrinol Metab. 2015;100:342–62.
19. Acosta A, Camilleri M, Abu Dayyeh B, Calderon G, Gonzalez D, McRae A, et al. Selection of antiobesity medications based on phenotypes enhances weight loss: a pragmatic trial in an obesity clinic. Obesity. 2021;29:662–71. The phenotype-guided (hungry brain (abnormal satiation), emotional hunger (hedonic eating), hungry gut (abnormal satiety), and slow burn (decreased metabolic rate) approach was associated with 1.75-fold greater weight loss after 12 months with mean weight loss of 15.9% compared with 9.0% in the non-phenotype-guided group–71.
20. Lau DCW, Erichsen L, Francisco AM, Satylganova A, le Roux CW, McGowan B, et al. Once-weekly cagrilintide for weight management in people with overweight and obesity: a multicentre, randomised, double-blind, placebo-controlled and active-controlled, dose-finding phase 2 trial. Lancet. 2021;398:2160–72.
21. Gibbons C, Blundell J, Tetens Hoff S, Dahl K, Bauer R, Bækdal T. Effects of oral semaglutide on energy intake, food preference, appetite, control of eating and body weight in subjects with type 2 diabetes. Diabetes Obes Metab. 2021,23.581–8.
22. Sorli C, Sichi H, Tsoukas GM, Unger J, Karsbøl JD, Hansen T, et al. Efficacy and safety of once-weekly semaglutide monotherapy versus placebo in patients with type 2 diabetes (SUSTAIN 1): a double-blind, randomised, placebo-controlled, parallel-group, multinational, multicentre phase 3a trial. Lancet Diabetes Endocrinol. 2017;5:251–60.
23. Ahrén B, Masmiquel L, Kumar H, Sargin M, Karsbøl JD, Jacobsen SH, et al. Efficacy and safety of once-weekly semaglutide versus once-daily sitagliptin as an add-on to metformin, thiazolidinediones, or both, in patients with type 2 diabetes (SUSTAIN 2): a 56-week, double-blind, phase 3a, randomised trial. Lancet Diabetes Endocrinol. 2017;5:341–54. https://pubmed.ncbi.nlm.nih.gov/28385659/
24. Ahmann AJ, Capehorn M, Charpentier G, Dotta F, Henkel E, Lingvay I, et al. Efficacy and safety of once-weekly semaglutide versus exenatide ER in subjects with type 2 diabetes (SUSTAIN 3): a 56-week, open-label randomized clinical trial. Diabetes Care. 2018;41:258–66.
25. Aroda VR, Bain SC, Cariou B, Piletič M, Rose L, Axelsen M, et al. Efficacy and safety of once-weekly semaglutide versus once-daily insulin glargine as add-on to metformin (with or without sulfonylureas) in insulin-naive patients with type 2 diabetes (SUSTAIN 4): a randomised, open-label, parallel-group, multicentre, multinational, phase 3a trial. Lancet Diabetes Endocrinol. 2017;5:355–66. https://doi.org/10.1016/S2213-8587(17)30085-2.
26. Rodbard HW, Lingvay I, Reed J, De La Rosa R, Rose L, Sugimoto D, et al. Semaglutide added to basal insulin in type 2 diabetes (SUSTAIN 5): a randomized, controlled trial. J Clin Endocrinol Metab. 2018;103:2291–301.

27. Pratley RE, Aroda VR, Lingvay I, Lüdemann J, Andreassen C, Navarria A, et al. Semaglutide versus dulaglutide once weekly in patients with type 2 diabetes (SUSTAIN 7): a randomised, open-label, phase 3b trial. Lancet Diabetes Endocrinol. 2018;6:275–86.
28. Thethi TK, Pratley R, Meier JJ. Efficacy, safety and cardiovascular outcomes of once-daily oral semaglutide in patients with type 2 diabetes: the PIONEER programme. Diabetes Obes Metab. 2020;22:1263–77.
29. Marso SP, Daniels GH, Brown-Frandsen K, Kristensen P, Mann JF, Nauck MA, et al. Liraglutide and cardiovascular outcomes in type 2 diabetes. N Engl J Med. 2016;375:311–22.
30. Marso SP, Bain SC, Consoli A, et al. Semaglutide and cardiovascular outcomes in patients with type 2 diabetes. N Engl J Med. 2016;375(19):1834–44.
31. Flint A, Andersen G, Hockings P, Johansson L, Morsing A, Sundby Palle M, et al. Randomised clinical trial: semaglutide versus placebo reduced liver steatosis but not liver stiffness in subjects with non-alcoholic fatty liver disease assessed by magnetic resonance imaging. Aliment Pharmacol Ther. 2021;54:1150–61.
32. Newsome NP, Buchholtz K, Cusi K, Linder M, Okanoue T, Ratziu V, et al. A placebo-controlled trial of subcutaneous semaglutide in nonalcoholic steatohepatitis. N Engl J Med. 2021;384:1113–24.
33. A Research Study on How Semaglutide Works in People With Fatty Liver Disease and Liver Damage - Full Text View - ClinicalTrials.gov. https://clinicaltrials.gov/ct2/show/NCT03987451.
34. Hartman ML, Sanyal AJ, Loomba R, Wilson JM, Nikooienejad A, Bray R, et al. Effects of novel dual GIP and GLP-1 receptor agonist tirzepatide on biomarkers of nonalcoholic steatohepatitis in patients with type 2. Diabetes Care. 2020;43:1352–5. https://pubmed.ncbi.nlm.nih.gov/32291277/
35. Blackman A, Foster GD, Zammit G, Rosenberg R, Aronne L, Wadden T, et al. Effect of liraglutide 3.0 mg in individuals with obesity and moderate or severe obstructive sleep apnea: the scale sleep apnea randomized clinical trial. Int J Obes. 2016;40:1310–9.
36. Obstructive Sleep Apnea Master Protocol GPIF: A Study of Tirzepatide (LY3298176) in Participants With Obstructive Sleep Apnea - Full Text View - ClinicalTrials.gov. https://clinicaltrials.gov/ct2/show/NCT05412004.
37. Deture MA, Dickson DW. The neuropathological diagnosis of Alzheimer's disease. Mol Neurodegener. 2019;14:32. https://doi.org/10.1186/s13024-019-0333-5.
38. Gejl M, Gjedde A, Egefjord L, Møller A, Hansen SB, Vang K, et al. In Alzheimer's disease, 6-month treatment with GLP-1 analog prevents decline of brain glucose metabolism: randomized, placebo-controlled, double-blind clinical trial. Front Aging Neurosci. 2016;8:108. https://doi.org/10.3389/fnagi.2016.00108.
39. Kalia LV, Lang AE. Parkinson's disease. Lancet. 2015;386(9996):896–912. https://doi.org/10.1016/S0140-6736(14)61393-3.
40. Pi-Sunyer X, Apovian CM, McElroy SL, Dunayevich E, Acevedo LM, Greenway FL. Psychiatric adverse events and effects on mood with prolonged-release naltrexone/bupropion combination therapy: a pooled analysis. Int J Obes. 2019;43:2085–94.
41. McElroy SL, Guerdjikova AI, Kim DD, et al. Naltrexone/bupropion combination therapy in overweight or obese patients with major depressive disorder: results of a pilot study. Prim Care Companion CNS Disord. 2013;15 https://doi.org/10.4088/PCC.12m01494.
42. Weina H, Yuhu N, Christian H, Birong L, Feiyu S, Le W. Liraglutide attenuates the depressive- and anxiety-like behaviour in the corticosterone induced depression model via improving hippocampal neural plasticity. Brain Res Brain Res. 2018;1694:55–62.
43. Seo MK, Jeong S, Seog DH, Lee JA, Lee JH, Lee Y, et al. Effects of liraglutide on depressive behavior in a mouse depression model and cognition in the probe trial of Morris water maze test. J Affect Disord. 2023;324:8–15.
44. Nedunchezhiyan U, Varughese I, Sun ARJ, Wu X, Crawford R, Prasadam I. Obesity, inflammation, and immune system in osteoarthritis. Front Immunol. 2022;13:907750. https://doi.org/10.3389/fimmu.2022.907750.

45. Gudbergsen H, Overgaard A, Henriksen M, Wæhrens EE, Bliddal H, Christensen R, et al. Liraglutide after diet-induced weight loss for pain and weight control in knee osteoarthritis: a randomized controlled trial. Am J Clin Nutr. 2021;113:314–23.
46. Research Study Looking at How Well Semaglutide Works in People Suffering From Obesity and Knee Osteoarthritis - ClinicalTrials.gov https://clinicaltrials.gov/ct2/show/NCT05064735.
47. Palmer MK, Toth PP. Trends in lipids, obesity, metabolic syndrome, and diabetes mellitus in the United States: an NHANES analysis (2003–2004 to 2013–2014). Obesity (Silver Spring). 2019;27(2):309–14.
48. Twig G, Yaniv G, Levine H, et al. Body-mass index in 2.3 million adolescents and cardiovascular death in adulthood. N Engl J Med. 2016;374(25):2430–40.
49. Powell-Wiley TM, Poirier P, Burke LE, et al. Obesity and cardiovascular disease: a scientific statement from the American Heart Association. Circulation. 2021;143:CIR0000000000000973.
50. Swift DL, McGee JE, Earnest CP, Carlisle E, Nygard M, Johannsen NM. The effects of exercise and physical activity on weight loss and maintenance. Prog Cardiovasc Dis. 2018;61(2):206–13.
51. Gibbs BB, Brancati FL, Chen H, et al. Effect of improved fitness beyond weight loss on cardiovascular risk factors in individuals with type 2 diabetes in the Look AHEAD study. Eur J Prev Cardiol. 2014;21(5):608–17.
52. Gorelik E, Gorelik B, Masarwa R, Perlman A, Hirsh-Raccah B, Matok I. The cardiovascular safety of antiobesity drugs-analysis of signals in the FDA Adverse Event Report System Database. Int J Obes. 2020;44(5):1021–7.
53. Glaysher MA, Ward J, Aldhwayan M, et al. The effect of a duodenal-jejunal bypass liner on lipid profile and blood concentrations of long chain polyunsaturated fatty acids. Clin Nutr. 2020;40:2343–54.
54. Fisher DP, Johnson E, Haneuse S, et al. Association between bariatric surgery and macrovascular disease outcomes in patients with type 2 diabetes and severe obesity. JAMA. 2018;320(15):1570–82.
55. Sjostrom L, Peltonen M, Jacobson P, Ahlin S, Andersson-Assarsson J, Anveden A, et al. Association of bariatric surgery with long-term remission of type 2 diabetes and with microvascular and macrovascular complications. JAMA. 2014;311(22):2297–304.
56. Eliasson B, Liakopoulos V, Franzen S, et al. Cardiovascular disease and mortality in patients with type 2 diabetes after bariatric surgery in Sweden: a nationwide, matched, observational cohort study. Lancet Diabetes Endocrinol. 2015;3(11):847–54.
57. Liakopoulos V, Franzen S, Svensson AM, et al. Renal and cardiovascular outcomes after weight loss from gastric bypass surgery in type 2 diabetes: cardiorenal risk reductions exceed atherosclerotic benefits. Diabetes Care. 2020;43(6):1276–84.
58. Moussa O, Ardissino M, Heaton T, et al. Effect of bariatric surgery on long-term cardiovascular outcomes: a nationwide nested cohort study. Eur Heart J. 2020;41(28):2660–7. Findings from this nested cohort study further evidenced that bariatric surgery not only improves CRF but also is associated with reduced CVD and death
59. Sheetz KH, Gerhardinger L, Dimick JB, Waits SA. Bariatric surgery and long-term survival in patients with obesity and end-stage kidney disease. JAMA Surg. 2020;155:581–8.
60. Blundell JE, Cooling J. Routes to obesity: phenotypes, food choices and activity. Br J Nutr. 2000;83(1):33–8.
61. Blundell JE, Stubs RJ, Golding C, et al. Resistance and susceptibility to weight gain: individual variability in response to a high-fat diet. Physiol Behav. 2005;86(5):614–22.
62. Nijs IM, Muris P, Euser AS, Franken IHA. Differences in attention to food and food intake between overweight/obese and normal-weight females under conditions of hunger and satiety. Appetite. 2010;54(2):243–54.
63. Massey A, Hill AJ. Dieting and food craving. A descriptive, quasi-prospective study. Appetite. 2012;58(3):781–5.
64. Warren C, Cooper PJ. Psychological effects of dieting. Br J Clin Psychol. 1988;27(3):269–70.

65. Keys A, Brožek J, Henschel A, Mickelsen O, Taylor HL. The biology of human starvation. (2 vols). University of Minnesota Press; 1950.
66. Welbourn R, Dixon J, Barth JH, et al. NICE-accredited commissioning guidance for weight assessment and management clinics: a model for a specialist multidisciplinary team approach for people with severe obesity. Obes Surg. 2016;26(3):649–59.
67. Horowitz M, Flint A, Jones KL, et al. Effect of the once-daily human GLP-1 analogue liraglutide on appetite, energy intake, energy expenditure and gastric emptying in type 2 diabetes. Diabetes Res Clin Pract. 2012;97(2):258–66.
68. Apovian CM, Aronne L, Rubino D, Still C, Wyatt H, Burns C, et al. A randomized, phase 3 trial of naltrexone SR/bupropion SR on weight and obesity-related risk factors (COR-II). Obesity (Silver Spring). 2013;21(5):935–43.
69. Khera R, Murad MH, Chandar AK, et al. Association of pharmacological treatments for obesity with weight loss and adverse events: a systematic review and meta-analysis. JAMA. 2016;315(22):2424–34.
70. Maayan L, Correll CU. Management of antipsychotic-related weight gain. Expert Rev Neurother. 2010;10(7):1175–200.
71. Fiedorowicz JG, Miller DD, Bishop JR, Calarge CA, Ellingrod VL, Haynes WG. Systematic review and meta-analysis of pharmacological interventions for weight gain from antipsychotics and mood stabilizers. Curr Psychiatr Rev. 2012;8(1):25–36.
72. Reekie J, Hosking SP, Prakash C, Kao KT, Juonala M, Sabin MA. The effect of antidepressants and antipsychotics on weight gain in children and adolescents. Obes Rev. 2015;16(7):566–80.
73. Larsen JR, Vedtofte L, Jakobsen MSL, Jespersen HR, Jakobsen MI, Svensson CK, et al. Effect of liraglutide treatment on prediabetes and overweight or obesity in clozapine- or olanzapine-treated patients with schizophrenia spectrum disorder: a randomized clinical trial. JAMA Psychiatry. 2017;74:719–28.
74. Zhuo C, Xu Y, Liu S, Li J, Zheng Q, Gao X, et al. Treatments in controlling antipsychotic-induced weight gain: a systematic review and network meta-analysis. Front Pharmacol. 2018a;28(9):1393.
75. Ellinger LK, Ipema HJ, Stachnik JM. Efficacy of metformin and topiramate in prevention and treatment of second-generation antipsychotic-induced weight gain. Ann Pharmacother. 2010;44(4):668–79.
76. Kendler KS, Gallagher TJ, Abelson JM. The National Comorbidity Survey: lifetime prevalence, demographic risk factors, and diagnostic validity of nonaffective psychosis as assessed in a US community sample. Arch Gen Psychiatry. 1996;53(11):1022–31.
77. Mizuno Y, Suzuki T, Nakagawa A, Yoshida K, Mimura M, Fleischhacker WW, et al. Pharmacological strategies to counteract antipsychotic-induced weight gain and metabolic adverse effects in schizophrenia: a systematic review and meta-analysis. Schizophr Bull. 2014;40(6):1385–403.
78. Ishøy PL, et al. Effect of GLP-1 receptor agonist treatment on body weight in obese antipsychotic-treated patients with schizophrenia: a randomized, placebo-controlled trial. Diabetes Obes Metab. 2017;19(2):162–71.
79. Siskind DJ, Russell AW, Gamble C, Winckel K, Mayfield K, et al. Treatment of clozapine-associated obesity and diabetes with exenatide in adults with schizophrenia: a randomized controlled trial (CODEX). Diabetes Obes Metab. 2018;20(4):1050–5.
80. Whicher CA, Price HC, Phiri P, Rathod S, Barnard-Kelly K, Reidy C, et al. Liraglutide and the management of overweight and obesity in people with schizophrenia, schizoaffective disorder and first-episode psychosis: protocol for a pilot trial. Trials Open access 20 November 2019. https://trialsjournal.biomedcentral.com/articles/10.1186/s13063-019-3689-5.
81. Whicher CA, Price HC, Phiri P, Rathod S, Barnard-Kelly K, Ngianga K, et al. The use of liraglutide 3.0mg daily in the management of overweight and obesity in people with schizophrenia, schozoaffective disorder and first episode psychosis: results of a pilot randomised double-blind placebo-controlled trial. Diabetes Obesity Metab. 2021;23:1262–71.

82. Aune D, Sen A, Prasad M, Norat T, Janszky I, Tonstad S, et al. BMI and all cause mortality: systematic review and non-linear dose-response meta-analysis of 230 cohort studies with 37.4 million deaths among 30.3 million participants. BMJ. 2016;353:2156.
83. James WPT, Caterson ID, Coutinho W, Finer N, Van Gaal LF, Maggioni AP, et al. Effect of sibutramine on cardiovascular outcomes in overweight and obese subjects. N Engl J Med. 2010;363:905–17.
84. Abbott Withdraws Sibutramine From Market [Internet]. [cited 2020]. Available from: https://www.medscape.com/viewarticle/730155.
85. Aagaard L, Hansen EH. Information about ADRs explored by pharmacovigilance approaches: a qualitative review of studies on antibiotics SSRIs and NSAIDs. BMC Clin Pharmacol. 2009;9:4.
86. Medications Target Long-Term Weight Control | FDA [Internet]. [cited 2021]. Available from: https://www.fda.gov/consumers/consumer-updates/medications-target-long-term-weight-control.
87. Ells LJ, et al. Interventions for treating children and adolescents with overweight and obesity: an overview of Cochrane reviews. Int J Obes. 2018;42:1823–33.
88. Wilding JPH, et al. Once-weekly semaglutide in adults with overweight or obesity. N Engl J Med. 2021;384:989–1002.
89. Wadden TA, et al. Effect of subcutaneous semaglutide vs placebo as an adjunct to intensive behavioral therapy on body weight in adults with overweight or obesity: the STEP 3 randomized clinical trial. JAMA J Am Med Assoc. 2021;325:1403–13.
90. Rubino D, et al. Effect of continued weekly subcutaneous semaglutide vs placebo on weight loss maintenance in adults with overweight or obesity: the STEP 4 randomized clinical trial. JAMA J Am Med Assoc. 2021;325:1414–25.
91. Rubino DM, et al. Effect of weekly subcutaneous semaglutide vs daily liraglutide on body weight in adults with overweight or obesity without diabetes: the STEP 8 randomized clinical trial. JAMA J Am Med Assoc. 2022;327:138–50.
92. Jebeile H, Kelly AS, O'Malley G, Baur LA. Obesity in children and adolescents: epidemiology, causes, assessment, and management. Lancet Diabetes Endocrinol. 2022;10:351–65.
93. Kelly AS, et al. Severe obesity in children and adolescents: identification, associated health risks, and treatment approaches: a scientific statement from the American Heart Association. Circulation. 2013;128:1689–712.
94. Ryder JR, Fox CK, Kelly AS. Treatment options for severe obesity in the pediatric population: current limitations and future opportunities. Obesity. 2018;26:951–60.
95. Hampl SE, et al. Clinical practice guideline for the evaluation and treatment of children and adolescents with obesity. Pediatrics. 2023;151:e2022060640.
96. Del Prato S, Gallwitz B, Holst JJ, Meier JJ. The incretin/glucagon system as a target for pharmacotherapy of obesity. Obes Rev. 2022;23:e13372.
97. Stumvoll M, Nurjhan N, Perriello G, Dailey G, Gerich JE. Metabolic effects of metformin in non-insulin-dependent diabetes mellitus. N Engl J Med. 1995;333(9):550–4.
98. D'Angelo MA, Raices M, Panowski SH, Hetzer MW. Age-dependent deterioration of nuclear pore complexes causes a loss of nuclear integrity in postmitotic cells. Cell. 2009;136(2):284–95.
99. Caprio S. Treatment of impaired glucose tolerance in childhood. Nat Clin Pract Endocrinol Metab. 2008;4:320–1.
100. Hearnshaw C, Matyka K. Managing childhood obesity: when lifestyle change is not enough. Diabetes Obes Metab. 2010;12:947–57.
101. Levri KM, et al. Metformin as treatment for overweight and obese adults: a systematic review. Ann Fam Med. 2005;3(5):457–61.
102. Park MH, Kinra S, Ward KJ, White B, Viner RM. Metformin for obesity in children and adolescents: a systematic review. Diabetes Care. 2009;32:1743–5.

103. Björkhem-Bergman L, Asplund AB, Lindh JD. Metformin for weight reduction in non-diabetic patients on antipsychotic drugs: a systematic review and meta-analysis. J Psychopharmacol. 2011;25:299–305.
104. McDonagh MS, Selph S, Ozpinar A, Foley C. Systematic review of the benefits and risks of metformin in treating obesity in children aged 18 years and younger. JAMA Pediatr. 2014;168:178–84.
105. Bouza C, López-Cuadrado T, Gutierrez-Torres LF, Amate J. Efficacy and safety of metformin for treatment of overweight and obesity in adolescents: an updated systematic review and meta-analysis. Obes Facts. 2012;5(5):753–65.
106. Desilets AR, Dhakal-Karki S, Dunican KC. Role of metformin for weight management in patients without type 2 diabetes. Ann Pharmacother. 2008;42:817–26.
107. Peirson L, Douketis J, Ciliska D, Fitzpatrick-Lewis D, Ali MU, Raina P. Treatment for overweight and obesity in adult populations: a systematic review and meta-analysis. CMAJ Open. 2014;2:E306–17.
108. Pasquali R, Gambineri A, Biscotti D, Vicennati V, Gagliardi L, Colitta D, Fiorini S, Cognigni GE, Filicori M, Morselli-Labate AM. Effect of long-term treatment with metformin added to hypocaloric diet on body composition, fat distribution, and androgen and insulin levels in abdominally obese women with and without the polycystic ovary syndrome. J Clin Endocrinol Metab. 2000;85:2767–74.
109. James AP, Watts GF, Mamo JCL. The effect of metformin and rosiglitazone on postprandial lipid metabolism in obese insulin-resistant subjects. Diabetes Obes Metab. 2005;7:381–9.
110. Kim C, Randolph JF, Golden SH, Labrie F, Kong S, Nan B, Barrett-Connor E. Weight loss decreases follicle stimulating hormone in overweight postmenopausal women. Obesity. 2015;23:228–33.
111. Lim SS, Norman RJ, Clifton PM, Noakes M. The effect of comprehensive lifestyle intervention or metformin on obesity in young women. Nutr Metab Cardiovasc Dis. 2011;21:261–8.
112. Pushpakom S, Iorio F, Eyers PA, Escott KJ, Hopper S, Wells A, et al. Drug repurposing: progress, challenges and recommendations. Nat Rev Drug Discov. 2019;18:41–58.
113. US FDA. Qsymia Prescribing Information (version 2012). 2012 [cited 2021 Jan 17]. Available at: https://www.accessdata.fda.gov/drugsatfda_docs/label/2012/022580s000lbl.pdf .
114. US FDA. Qsymia Approval Letter. 2012 [cited 2021 Jan 17]. Available at: https://www.accessdata.fda.gov/drugsatfda_docs/appletter/2012/022580Origs000ltr.pdf.
115. Chen C-Y, Bussing R, Hartzema AG, Shuster JJ, Segal R, Winterstein AG. Stimulant use following the publicity of cardiovascular safety and the introduction of patient medication guides. Pharmacoepidemiol Drug Saf. 2016;25:678–86.
116. Bessesen DH, Van Gaal LF. Progress and challenges in anti-obesity pharmacotherapy. Lancet Diabetes Endocrinol. 2018;6(3):237–48.
117. Sarayani A, Albogami Y, Thai TN, Smolinski NE, Patel P, Wang Y, et al. Prenatal exposure to teratogenic medications in the era of risk evaluation and mitigation strategies. Am J Obstet Gynecol. 2022;227:263.e1–263.e38.
118. Druce M, Bloom SR. Central regulators of food intake. Curr Opin Clin Nutr Metab Care. 2003;6:361–7.
119. Halford JC, Cooper GD, Dovey TM. The pharmacology of human appetite expression. Curr Drug Targets. 2004;5:221–40.
120. Rushing PA, Hagan MM, Seeley RJ, Lutz TA, Woods SC. Amylin: a novel action in the brain to reduce body weight. Endocrinology. 2000;141:850–3.
121. Reidelberger RD, Haver AC, Arnelo U, Smith DD, Schaffert CS, Permert J. Amylin receptor blockade stimulates food intake in rats. Am J Phys. 2004;287:R568–74.
122. Maggs DG, Fineman MS, Kornstein J, et al. Pramlintide reduces postprandial glucose excursions when added to insulin lispro in subjects with type 2 diabetes: a dose timing study. Diabetes Metab Res Rev. 2004;20:55–60.
123. Vella A, Lee JS, Camilleri M, et al. Effects of pramlintide, an amylin analogue, on gastric emptying in type 1 and 2 diabetes mellitus. Neurogastroenterol Motil. 2002;14:123–31.

124. Després JP, Lemieux I, Prud'homme D. Treatment of obesity: need to focus on high risk abdominally obese patients. BMJ. 2001;322(7288):716–20.
125. Rosenbaum M, Hirsch J, Gallagher DA, Leibel RL. Long-term persistence of adaptive thermogenesis in subjects who have maintained a reduced body weight. Am J Clin Nutr. 2008;88(4):906–12.
126. Grunvald E, Shah R, Hernaez R, Chandar AK, Pickett-Blakely O, Teigen LM, et al. AGA clinical practice guideline on pharmacological interventions for adults with obesity. Gastroenterology. 2022;163(5):1198–225.
127. Saxenda (liraglutide) [package insert]. Plainsboro, NJ: Novo Nordisk; 2020.
128. Rubino D, Abrahamsson N, Davies M, et al. Effect of continued weekly subcutaneous semaglutide vs placebo on weight loss maintenance in adults with overweight or obesity: the STEP 4 randomized clinical trial. JAMA. 2021;325(14):1414–25.
129. Wadden TA, Bailey TS, Billings LK, et al. Effect of subcutaneous semaglutide vs placebo as an adjunct to intensive behavioral therapy on body weight in adults with overweight or obesity: the STEP 3 randomized clinical trial. JAMA. 2021;325(14):1403–13.
130. Wilding JPH, Batterham RL, Calanna S, et al. Once-weekly semaglutide in adults with overweight or obesity. N Engl J Med. 2021;384(11):989–1002.
131. Davies M, Færch L, Jeppesen OK, et al. Semaglutide 2·4 mg once a week in adults with overweight or obesity, and type 2 diabetes (STEP 2): a randomised, double-blind, double-dummy, placebo-controlled, phase 3 trial. Lancet. 2021;397(10278):971–84.
132. Rosenstock J, Wysham C, Frías JP, Kaneko S, Lee CJ, Fernández Landó L, et al. Efficacy and safety of a novel dual GIP and GLP-1 receptor agonist tirzepatide in patients with type 2 diabetes (SURPASS-1): a double-blind, randomised, phase 3 trial [published correction appears in Lancet. 2021 Jul 17;398(10296):212]. Lancet. 2021;398:143–55.
133. Frías JP, Davies MJ, Rosenstock J, Pérez Manghi FC, Fernández Landó L, Bergman BK, et al. Tirzepatide versus semaglutide once weekly in patients with type 2 diabetes. N Engl J Med. 2021;385:503–15.
134. Jastreboff AM, Aronne LJ, Ahmad NN, Wharton S, Connery L, Alves B, et al. Tirzepatide once weekly for the treatment of obesity. N Engl J Med. 2022;387:205–16.
135. Ambery P, Parker VE, Stumvoll M, Posch MG, Heise T, Plum-Moerschel L, et al. MEDI0382, a GLP-1 and glucagon receptor dual agonist, in obese or overweight patients with type 2 diabetes: a randomised, controlled, double-blind, ascending dose and phase 2a study. Lancet. 2018;391(10140):2607–18.
136. Di Prospero NA, Yee J, Frustaci ME, Samtani MN, Alba M, Fleck P. Efficacy and safety of glucagon-like peptide-1/glucagon receptor co-agonist JNJ-64565111 in individuals with type 2 diabetes mellitus and obesity: a randomized dose-ranging study. Clin Obes. 2021;11:e12433.
137. Klein S, JJ N Jr, Harris MS, Suyundikov A, Casper R, Steele SM, et al. 334-OR: Pemvidutide (ALT-801), a balanced (1:1) GLP-1/glucagon dual receptor agonist, induces rapid and marked weight loss without the need for dose titration in people with overweight/obesity. Diabetes. 2022;71(Suppl_1)
138. Urva S, Coskun T, Loh MT, Du Y, Thomas MK, Gurbuz S, et al. LY3437943, a novel triple GIP, GLP-1, and glucagon receptor agonist in people with type 2 diabetes: a phase 1b, multicentre, double-blind, placebo-controlled, randomised, multiple-ascending dose trial. Lancet. 2022;400:1869–81.
139. Calderon G, Gonzalez-Izundegui D, Shan KL, Garcia-Valencia OA, Cifuentes L, Campos A, Collazo-Clavell ML, Shah M, Hurley DL, Abu Lebdeh HS, Sharma M, Schmitz K, Clark MM, Grothe K, Mundi MS, Camilleri M, Abu Dayyeh BK, Hurtado Andrade MD, Mokadem MA, Acosta A. Effectiveness of anti-obesity medications approved for long-term use in a multidisciplinary weight management program: a multi-center clinical experience. Int J Obes. 2021;46:555–63. https://doi.org/10.1038/s41366-021-01019-6.

140. Guglielmi V, Bettini S, Sbraccia P, Busetto L, Pellegrini M, Yumuk V, Colao AM, El Ghoch M, Muscogiuri G. Beyond weight loss: added benefits could guide the choice of anti-obesity medications. Curr Obes Rep. 2023;12:127–46. https://doi.org/10.1007/s13679-023-00502-7.
141. Iwamoto SJ, Abushamat LA, Zaman A, Millard AJ, Cornier M-A. Obesity management in cardiometabolic disease: state of the art. Curr Atheroscler Rep. 2021;23:59. https://doi.org/10.1007/s11883-021-00953-0.
142. Roberts CA, Christiansen P, Halford JCG. Tailoring pharmacotherapy to specific eating behaviours in obesity: can recommendations for personalised therapy be made from the current data? Acta Diabetol. 2017;54:715–25. https://doi.org/10.1007/s00592-017-0994-x.
143. Wang C, Shi W, Xu J, Huang C, Zhu J. Outcomes and safety of concomitant topiramate or metformin for antipsychotics-induced obesity: a randomized-controlled trial. Ann General Psychiatry. 2020;19:68. https://doi.org/10.1186/s12991-020-00319-x.
144. Barnard-Kelly K, Whicher CA, Price HC, Phiri P, Rathod S, Asher C, Peveler RC, Holt RIG. Liraglutide and the management of overweight and obesity in people with severe mental illness: qualitative sub-study. BMC Psychiatry. 2022;22:21. https://doi.org/10.1186/s12888-021-03666-5.
145. Alsuhibani A, Alrasheed M, Gari M, Hincapie AL, Guo JJ. Descriptive analysis of reported adverse events associated with anti-obesity medications using FDA Adverse Event Reporting System (FAERS) databases 2013–2020. Int J Clin Pharm. 2021;44:172–9. https://doi.org/10.1007/s11096-021-01330-2.
146. Kelly AS. Current and future pharmacotherapies for obesity in children and adolescents. Nat Rev Endocrinol. 2023;19:534–41. https://doi.org/10.1038/s41574-023-00858-9.
147. Yerevanian A, Soukas AA. Metformin: mechanisms in human obesity and weight loss. Curr Obes Rep. 2019;8:156–64. https://doi.org/10.1007/s13679-019-00335-3.
148. Hui F, Zhang Y, Ren T, Li X, Zhao M, Zhao Q. Role of metformin in overweight and obese people without diabetes: a systematic review and network meta-analysis. Eur J Clin Pharmacol. 2018;75:437–50. https://doi.org/10.1007/s00228-018-2593-3.
149. Sarayani A, Hampp C, Brown JD, Donahoo WT, Winterstein AG. Topiramate utilization after phentermine/Topiramate approval for obesity management: risk minimization in the era of drug repurposing. Drug Saf. 2022;45:1517–27. https://doi.org/10.1007/s40264-022-01244-6.
150. Chapman I, Parker B, Doran S, Feinle-Bisset C, Wishart J, Strobel S, Wang Y, Burns C, Lush C, Weyer C, Horowitz M. Effect of pramlintide on satiety and food intake in obese subjects and subjects with type 2 diabetes. Diabetologia. 2005;48:838–48. https://doi.org/10.1007/s00125-005-1732-4.
151. Schmitz S, Tchang BG, Shukla AP. Obesity pharmacotherapy: a review of current practices and future directions. Curr Treat Options Gastroenterol. 2023;21:27–47. https://doi.org/10.1007/s11938-023-00409-1.